# Academic General Practice in the UK Medical Schools, 1948–2000

A Short History

Edited by John Howie and
Michael Whitfield

Edinburgh University Press

© in this edition Edinburgh University Press, 2011
© in the individual contributions is retained by the authors

Edinburgh University Press Ltd
22 George Square, Edinburgh

www.euppublishing.com

Typeset in 10.5/13 pt Adobe Sabon
by Servis Filmsetting Ltd, Stockport, Cheshire, and
printed and bound in Great Britain by
CPI Antony Rowe, Chippenham and Eastbourne

A CIP record for this book is available from the British Library

ISBN 978 0 7486 4356 1 (paperback)

The right of the contributors
to be identified as author of this work
has been asserted in accordance with
the Copyright, Designs and Patents Act 1988.

# Contents

*Preface*

Imagine a country whose medical schools do not systematically teach students within the clinical discipline that most of them would work in. Imagine such a country also failing to conduct research into the clinical and organisational problems faced by patients and the doctors working in that discipline. Although it seems unthinkable now, the UK was such a country when the NHS began. This book describes and analyses how the pioneers of academic general practice in the UK and the Republic of Ireland overcame the challenges and obstacles to achieving their vision of ensuring that all undergraduates in every medical school experience excellent education in a research-rich environment.

The editors have compiled chapters from departments across the country, telling the highly variable story about how each made progress within their own context. Support from postgraduate departments, the RCGP, departments of public health and parts of the NHS all played their part. The appendices describe the new medical schools; the crucial SIFT/ACT developments; an integrating perspective; and the transition from AUTGP to AUDGP to SAPC. For many readers the main interest will lie in the story of their own institution but others will see common themes and insights that will help them understand how support for progress can be marshalled within and across organisations to overcome today's challenges.

The main part of the story told here ends in 2000. However the subsequent decade has confirmed the solidity of the foundations laid by the earlier pioneers. No one in the UK now questions the need for academic general practice to be a major part of the undergraduate medical curriculum, and primary care is seen as one of the country's key research strengths. General practitioners no longer work only in departments of general practice but have joined, and lead, a wide range of other academic groups. The next generation are also reaching out to other countries who want to develop the kinds of benefits from teaching and research we now consider normal.

*Frank Sullivan*
*Chair, Heads of Departments Group SAPC*

# Acknowledgements

The editors wish to thank all who have contributed material for the twenty-one chapters and four appendices which make up this history, most but not all of whom are named in the appropriate places. Their support has mirrored the consistently collegiate ethos which has been the hallmark of our community over the years. Without their hard work and willingness to respond quickly to requests for help, the final story would have been far less complete and much less interesting. Roger Jones commented valuably on a late edition of the manuscript, and George Freeman was particularly helpful in the collation of several of the London histories.

We are particularly grateful to David Weller who made funding available from the James Mackenzie Fund to enable this work to be published, and to Jackie Jones and her staff at Edinburgh University Press for their enthusiastic support at all stages of its production.

Finally we thank the Editor of the *British Journal of General Practice* for permission to reproduce Appendix 3.

# *Abbreviations*

| | |
|---|---|
| ACT | Addition for Clinical Teaching |
| ASM | Annual Scientific Meeting |
| AUDGP | Association of University Departments of General Practice |
| AUDGPI | Association of University Teachers of General Practice in Ireland |
| AUPMC | Academic Unit of Primary Medical Care |
| AUTGP | Association of University Teachers of General Practice |
| | |
| BJGP | British Journal of General Practice |
| BMA | British Medical Association |
| | |
| CBT | Community Based Teaching |
| CMO | Chief Medical Officer |
| CSO | Chief Scientist Organisation |
| CPSE | Clinical and Population Sciences and Education |
| | |
| DH | Department of Health |
| DHSS | Department of Health and Social Services |
| | |
| EGPRW | European General Practice Research Workshop |
| EU | European Union |
| | |
| FBA | Fellowship by Assessment |
| FHSA | Family Health Services Authority |
| | |
| GMC | General Medical Council |
| GMSC | General Medical Services Committee |
| GPRN | General Practice Research Network |
| GPTU | General Practice Teaching Unit |
| GPU | General Practice Unit |

| | |
|---|---|
| HEFC | Higher Education Funding Council |
| HRB | Health Research Board |
| HSR | Health Services Research |
| | |
| ICRF | Imperial Cancer Research Fund |
| | |
| JCPTGP | Joint Committee on Postgraduate Training for General Practice |
| JRCGP | Journal of the Royal College of General Practitioners |
| | |
| LATS | London Academic Trainee Scheme |
| LIZEI | London Implementation Zone Educational Initiatives |
| LMC | Local Medical Committee |
| | |
| MRC | Medical Research Council |
| | |
| NAPCRG | North American Primary Care Research Group |
| NHS | National Health Service |
| NIHR | National Institute of Health Research |
| NPCRDC | National Primary Care Research and Development Centre |
| | |
| OSCE | Objective Structured Clinical Examination |
| | |
| PCRN | Primary Care Research Network |
| PCT | Primary Care Trust |
| PES | Public Expenditure Settlement |
| PMO | Principal Medical Officer |
| PPD | Personal and Professional Development |
| | |
| QAA | Quality Assurance Agency |
| QOF | Quality and Outcomes Framework |
| | |
| R&D | Research and Development |
| RAE | Research Assessment Exercise |
| RAWP | Resource Allocation Working Party |
| RCGP | Royal College of General Practitioners |
| RHA | Regional Health Authority |
| RSU | Research Support Unit |
| | |
| SAPC | Society of Academic Primary Care |
| SGUMDER | Standing Group on Medical and Dental Education and Research |

| | |
|---|---|
| SHHD | Scottish Home and Health Department |
| SIFT | Service Increment For Teaching |
| SIMG | Societas Internationalis Medicinae Generalis |
| SSPC | Scottish School of Primary Care |
| StaRNeT | South Thames Primary Care Network |
| | |
| UGC | University Grants Committee |
| UMDS | United Medical and Dental Schools |
| | |
| WONCA | World Organization of National Colleges, Academies and Academic Associations of General Practitioners/Family Physicians |

# Timeline

| First funded undergraduate general practice academic post | Other significant events |
|---|---|
| 1948 Edinburgh | |
| 1965 Manchester | |
| 1966 | 'GP Charter' |
| 1967 Aberdeen, St Thomas's | |
| 1968 Cardiff, Guy's, Southampton | |
| 1969 Newcastle | |
| 1970 Dundee | |
| 1971 Belfast, Liverpool, St Mary's, UCL | |
| 1972 Glasgow, Sheffield, Nottingham | first ASM, Cardiff |
| 1973 Trinity College Dublin | |
| 1974 Birmingham, Leeds | |
| 1975 Leicester | |
| 1976 Cambridge | |
| 1977 Charing Cross, Oxford | |
| 1978 George's, King's | |
| 1981 Middlesex | |

| | | |
|---|---|---|
| 1983 | | Guy's + St Thomas's merged as UMDS |
| 1984 | | Westminster + Charing Cross |
| 1985 | | Middlesex + University College |
| 1986 | Bristol, Royal Free | |
| 1987 | Royal College of Surgeons in Ireland | St Mary's + Imperial |
| 1990 | | Fund-holding |
| 1991 | UC Dublin | |
| 1992 | | SIFT/ACT available |
| 1993 | | GMC Tomorrow's Doctors |
| 1994 | | Royal Free + UCL |
| 1995 | | St Bartholomew's + The London + Queen Mary and Westfield |
| 1997 | UC Cork, NUI Galway, Warwick | Charing Cross + Imperial |
| 1998 | | UMDS + King's |
| 2001 | Keele | |
| 2002 | Hull York, Peninsula, East Anglia | |
| 2003 | Brighton and Sussex | |
| 2004 | Swansea | |
| 2007 | Limerick | |
| 2008 | St Andrews | |

# Introduction

In July 2007, the Heads of Departments group of SAPC invited those of their retired predecessors and founder members of AUTGP they could trace to join them for their annual get-together in an Indian restaurant in South Kensington. Anxious to repay their hospitality and recognising that many of our stories of the early struggles and setbacks along the road to where we were now had never been properly recorded and were in danger of being lost, our cluster of veterans agreed to write about the early developments of our respective departments. Four years on, this book is the result.

Predictably, our writers did not want to be constrained by any particular format, although we originally signed up to a target length of around 1,000 words. At the end of two years we had six essays in; twenty-five to come! A number of founder heads were no longer with us, or no longer able to contribute, so we set about finding deputies. The original London schools proved a particular challenge, having been so complicated by later mergers and their earliest roots often hard to trace. Some of our most compelling essays have been written in the first person, but most are in the third person. Some were well over our target length; in some we identified important gaps; and some were referenced although most were not. Most problematically, some were concluded (naturally on the retirement of the author) in the late 1970s or early 1980s before other stories had started.

The common denominators within the essays are the strong vision and tenacity of our early academic leaders, the key support of a few established academics (more often than not professors of public health), the equally critical obstruction from senior establishment figures whose help would have made all the difference (although these are played down by most of our authors), the substantial and critical support from local general practitioners, and the struggle to identify even minimal funding to support early academic developments. So critical was the arrival of

SIFT/ACT money in 1993 (described in our second appendix) that we decided that while keeping our focus on the early events in our histories, we would try to capture at least in outline events up to 2000. This has also allowed us to better reflect the hugely important role played by social scientists in our evolution across the decades. In the end, at the request of the current Heads of Departments, we have now added updates on still more recent events, these highlighting a trend back to unions with departments we had spent so much earlier effort trying to gain independence from. But we have kept our title dates to our original choice of 1948 to 2000 as it is the story of these early achievements we wanted this volume to celebrate in particular.

Our referees and sponsors suggested we include predictions about the future and include an international perspective, but these were not our original purposes. However, we have included four appendices, one about the new medical schools developed since 2000, and one about how SAPC has progressed in the years since 2000 when it replaced the AUDGP, signalling the progressive evolution of the discipline of academic general practice to that of academic primary care. The third describes the story of the SIFT/ACT negotiations which unlocked the critical funding stream whose value is so evident throughout our collection of essays; our fourth appendix presents one attempt to put our history within a more analytical framework.

Two things to end with. First, our sincere thanks to the many colleagues – both retired and still actively working – whose efforts have made this publication possible; many are identified as authors, but others have helped in materially important ways as well. Second, we have struggled to find a catchy title which properly captures what this history is about. What we have settled on may not excite at first glance, but it does describe what has been the major concern of our project. The story of academic general practice has been one of solid achievement, slow at first but then with steadily increasing momentum and impact to the position of substantial achievement so clearly recorded in the pages which follow. We hope that our narrative will inform and inspire the next telling of the story, whenever that may be and whatever may be its title.

*John Howie, Edinburgh*
*Michael Whitfield, Bristol*
*December 2010*

Without memories there are no images

Without images the existence of man,
of a generation, of a people, cannot be collected,
recognized, or communicated

*Museo Agricola el Patio*
*Tiagua, Lanzarote*

# Chapter 1

# The University of Aberdeen

Aberdeen students in the pre-NHS era received an introduction to general practice during attachments to the Woolmanhill public dispensary as part of their public health teaching. Between 1948 and the creation of the GPTU in 1967, there was no formal teaching in general practice, although many students fixed up short attachments to north-east general practices on their own initiative during vacations.

## 1967–1984

In 1967, with a grant from the Nuffield Provincial Hospitals Trust, the university decided to create the GPTU and advertised for a director at senior lecturer/reader level. Forty-four applications were received, the majority from senior north-east general practitioners without academic experience. Applicants from outside the area included several already in academic general practice positions. Ian Richardson was appointed from the local department of public health, bringing to the position substantial intellectual skills and a strong academic record in the field of community-based teaching and research.

His appointment heralded the start of a period of substantial and sustained achievement. An undergraduate programme dependent on significant good will from practices throughout the north-east of Scotland was developed, as was Aberdeen's vocational training scheme which, with twelve places each year, was the largest of its kind in the UK. With Ian Buchan, Ian Richardson carried out a major time-and-motion study of the general practice consultation, an idea later repeated for district nurses and health visitors.

The department achieved independent status in 1970 when the chair in general practice was established, supported by the residue of the James Mackenzie money which had been used to create the Edinburgh chair in 1963. The Aberdeen department was the first to be wholly funded with UGC money as against relying on NHS income from general practice work. The absence of formal staff contracts to provide patient care was both a strength and a weakness. A weakness in so far as it attracted questions about the department's clinical credibility, but a strength in terms of the time it made available to develop teaching and research programmes.

John Howie was the first new full-time academic appointment, with research interests in decision-making in respiratory illnesses and anti-biotic use, followed by John Berkeley (cottage hospitals), Ross Taylor (pre- and post-menopausal symptoms) and John Bain (otitis media). Six local general practitioners (Denis Durno, Pierre Fouin, Alec Taylor, Geoffrey Gill, Fraser Richardson and James Shand) were given part-time lecturer contracts, contributing materially to the balance of the depart-ment. In the late 1970s, Denis Durno became regional adviser in general practice for the north-east of Scotland.

The department was originally housed in a hut within the back car park of Aberdeen Royal Infirmary at Foresterhill. One of Ian Richardson's significant early research projects had involved mapping a health centre plan for the city of Aberdeen, including a teaching health centre within the Foresterhill campus. This was realised in 1977, the department being embedded alongside three working practices, in each of which one of the full-time lecturers had a clinical attachment.

In 1980, Ian Richardson became the first UK general practice aca-demic to become Dean of a faculty of medicine, but his deanship was made difficult by its coinciding with the 'volume cuts' of the period, which saw 24 per cent cut from university budgets over a three-year time frame. John Howie and John Bain left to take up chairs in Edinburgh and Southampton, and John Berkeley to an NHS administrative post, none of their positions being replaced. Two part-time lecturers were appointed (Michael Taylor and Lewis Ritchie). Ian Richardson took early retirement in 1984, and his post too was frozen. A period of difficulty and retrenchment was to follow.

## 1984–1992

Following Ian Richardson's retirement, Roy Weir, who was profes-sor of community medicine, became acting head of department, with Ross Taylor continuing as the only full-time clinical academic. An unsuccessful public appeal was made to raise funds to re-establish the James Mackenzie chair. In 1988, Ross Taylor was appointed senior lecturer and head of department. With the support of his part-time lecturer colleagues, he laid the foundations for the re-establishment of the Mackenzie chair in 1992. During this difficult period, Ross steadfastly led a significant increase in teaching and research activity, grant income gained, and the appointment of new research personnel, including expertise in pharmacy and clinical psychology. During this period, the regional adviser's unit relocated away from the Foresterhill Health Centre, Denis Durno retired and was succeeded by Bill Reith.

## 1992–2010

Following his appointment as Dean of Medicine, Professor (later Sir) Graeme Catto re-established the Mackenzie chair with funding support from Grampian Health Board and Lewis Ritchie was appointed. Like Ian Richardson, Lewis had a background in both public health and general practice, and he continued to practise clinical medicine at Peterhead. The department underwent substantial expansion, developing research themes including cardiovascular disease prevention, computing/telemedicine, oncology, medicines management/prescribing, women's health (oral contraception), primary care epidemiology, substance misuse, and rural health. Teaching commitments increased threefold in response to the 1993 GMC document *Tomorrow's Doctors*. In 1996, a key development was the endowment by the local health board of a second professorial chair, the NHS Grampian research chair of primary care. In 1997 Philip Hannaford became first incumbent, moving from his position as director of the RCGP epidemiology unit in Manchester and relocating the oral contraception study that had originally been established there by Clifford Kay.

In 1966, the department changed its name to the department of general practice and primary care, recognising the increasingly multidisciplinary nature of service general practice and primary care. In 1998, the Centre for Advanced Studies in Nursing became co-located in the department, and was subsequently assimilated within it. Christine Bond became the third professor in the department when she was promoted to a personal chair in primary care pharmacy in 1999. The same year, as part of a combined initiative involving all four Scottish departments of general practice, Lewis Ritchie led the inauguration and initial fund raising for the Scottish School of Primary Care, which aimed to increase primary care research capacity and quality in Scotland. A fourth chair followed, in 2000, when David Price was appointed to the General Practice Airways Group chair of primary care respiratory medicine. Since 2000, two further personal chairs have been appointed (Amanda Lee in statistics, and Blair Smith in primary care medicine), and the department has become one of the largest departments of general practice in the UK. In the 2001 RAE, Aberdeen joined Birmingham, Cambridge, Manchester and Oxford as one of the top rated UK departments of general practice.

In 2007, Lewis Ritchie stepped down as head of the department of general practice and primary care. The department was renamed the Centre of Academic Primary Care (CAPC) as part of an internal school of medicine restructuring into divisions and sections. Christine Bond was appointed as section leader, and the Centre for Rural Health at Inverness (whose director was Professor David Godden) was also assimilated as part of CAPC.

*Lewis Ritchie*
*John Howie*

# Chapter 2

# The University of Dundee

Dundee is a small Scottish city with one of the smaller medical schools in the UK. Academic general practice has played an important role in its contribution to medical education and, increasingly, research.

## The early years: 1970–1992

The University of Dundee began as a college of the University of St Andrews and became an independent institution in 1967. The senior faculty of its medical school soon realised it needed a department of general practice. On 1 April 1970, Dr James Knox left his practice in Edinburgh to become the inaugural professor of general practice.

Originally based near the main university campus in the centre of the city, but remote from the medical school at Ninewells Hospital, the department was without a clinical base. Early priorities included identifying a cadre of general practitioner contributors to the undergraduate teaching programme, working on content, teaching and assessment methods in a programme of problem-based learning, and helping the new tutors to acquire the necessary skills to fulfil their tasks. Contrary to expectations in some quarters within the university, the department's teaching was not 'more of the same', but was breaking new ground. Throughout the ensuing years, a feature of the department's activities was arranging frequent meetings with general practitioners in many different (usually informal) settings.

### Research

The Scottish General Practitioner Research Support Unit (RSU) was a medium-term project intended to assist general practitioners locally and nationally to develop their own research ideas in their own practices. The collaboration involved the University of Dundee, the RCGP and the SHHD CSO. The RSU functioned successfully between 1970 and 1980 by which time all Scottish medical schools had their own departments of general practice.

Initially the RSU's activities were supervised by a board, chaired by the late W. Gregson of Ferranti in Edinburgh, which met two or three times a year, but later the SHHD took over this role. The RSU closed in 1980 after a decade of providing encouragement, advice and statistical help to numerous doctors throughout Scotland, assisting them in studies, some for higher degrees. It provided a base for a large study, led by Albert Jacob, a Dundee general practitioner, into the effects of new health centres on Dundee's primary health care. It also ran an influenza monitoring service involving fifty Tayside general practitioners.

## Teaching

It was seven years before the medical school teaching practice was established with its own list of 2,000 patients based in the Westgate Health Centre in the grounds of Ninewells Hospital – the first example of a general practice teaching and research facility based in such close proximity to the traditional focus of medical teaching. The development owed much to Campbell Murdoch (senior lecturer) and lecturers Peter Campion and Ron Neville. Eventually Professor Knox joined the practice as a principal.

The main aim of the department was to complement hospital-based medical teaching by using the setting of general practice for student learning. Emphasis was put on problem solving. One particular role assumed by the department and shared with others (notably the behavioural scientists), was helping students to acquire and enhance their interviewing skills. This was introduced to students in the pre-clinical phase, and involved the use of both real patients and actors and the use of video-feedback. Another contribution was the development of problem-based assessment using various methods, including the modified essay question.

## Tayside centre for general practice (TCGP): 1992

In 1992 John Bain was appointed as Professor Knox's successor. Like Professor Knox, he had been a trainee in the department of general

practice in Edinburgh with Professor Richard Scott. He had also held
the chair of general practice in Southampton before moving to Dundee.
When he arrived discussions began with the postgraduate department
led by Robin Scott to create an integrated unit. The acquisition of funds
from the Scottish Office for new purpose-built premises allowed the
creation of the TCGP.[1] This innovative development, the first in the
UK, achieved many of its original aims, including promoting primary
care research, facilitating audit through the Tayside Audit Resource for
Primary Care, supporting practice development, and developing undergraduate and postgraduate education in general practice and career
opportunities for general practice researchers, teachers and trainers.

This was the prelude to further expansion and the creation of the
Mackenzie Building which now houses general practice, public health
medicine, the drugs surveillance unit, and the dental health research
unit. This has allowed collaborative research which has enhanced the
standing of primary care research in Dundee.

Once these major changes in learning and professional development
were well established, NHS Tayside agreed to create a chair of research
and development in general practice and primary care. Frank Sullivan
moved from the University of Glasgow to take up this post. As John
Bain neared retirement in 2001, Dave Snadden, now regional adviser,
became head of TCGP. Dave initiated the multi-institutional Scottish
MSc in primary care which continues to provide Masters training across
a range of primary care disciplines in Scotland.[2] When John Bain retired,
Tom Fahey joined TCGP from Bristol as professor of primary care medicine. Four years later, when he moved to Dublin, his place was taken
by Bruce Guthrie, returning to Scotland from a Harkness Fellowship in
Stanford, USA.


## Divisionalisation: 2005

In recent years departments have become unfashionable management
entities and the University of Dundee has followed the trend. Academic
general practice in Dundee plays a major role in the new division of
Clinical and Population Sciences and Education (CPSE) of the College
of Medicine, Dentistry and Nursing as well as in the East of Scotland
postgraduate deanery. Led by Jon Dowell (reader), undergraduate education in the early years is integrated with teaching in communication
skills, clinical skills, public health and behavioural science. In later years
students are taught in practices all over Scotland and in the innovative
Medicine in Malawi Project. The postgraduate director for the East of

Scotland deanery is currently David Bruce, and continuing professional development is being led by Mairi Scott in the Professional Development Academy. Within Dundee our research is increasingly focused on issues of quality, safety and informatics with Bruce Guthrie leading the multi-disciplinary group of that name in CPSE. Other research is co-ordinated by the Scottish School of Primary Care whose current director is Frank Sullivan.[3]

Dundee's particular strength has been the people of Dundee and Tayside who have tolerated and now welcome medical students from around the world. They are also enthusiastic partners helping us to address research questions. Building on the foundations of earlier years, TCGP continues to work across the full academic spectrum.

*James Knox*
*Frank Sullivan*

## Notes

1. Bain J., Scott R. and Snadden D., 'Integrating undergraduate and postgraduate education in general practice: experience in Tayside', *BMJ*, 310, 1995: 1577–79.
2. Scottish MSc in Primary Care: http://www.sspc.ac.uk/mscprimarycare
3. The Scottish School of Primary Care: http://www.sspc.ac.uk

# Chapter 3

# The University of Edinburgh

During the second half of the eighteenth century, Andrew Duncan – then professor of medicine in the University of Edinburgh – proposed and constructed a public dispensary to provide care to the sick poor in the Old Town of Edinburgh and to instruct medical students. From 1890 attendance at one of several public dispensary practices became a compulsory part of the Edinburgh undergraduate curriculum.[1]

As in many UK medical schools, the development of the academic department owed much to the foresight and opportunism of senior academic public health/social medicine physicians. In Edinburgh, Professor Frank Crew recognised that the closure of the public dispensaries at the start of the NHS in 1948 would be an important loss to the education of medical students. In 1947, Richard Scott, then a lecturer in Crew's department and with pre-war experience in general practice, embarked on a project to explore the medical and social needs of families in sickness and in health, and together they sought to establish a 'laboratory in the community' to provide teaching to medical students and for long-term studies of illness within families.

So, on the first day of the NHS in July 1948, Richard Scott together with a medical assistant, an almoner, a nurse and a dentist set up an NHS practice within the Royal Public Dispensary in West Richmond Street. By 1951 some thirty medical students each year were being provided with a three-month course of clinical instruction, and in 1952 the Rockefeller Foundation offered financial support to aid the development of general practice as an academic discipline. With that support, the West Richmond Street practice joined the Livingstone Memorial Dispensary in the Cowgate to form the General Practice Teaching Unit. In 1956 the GPTU was given independent status as the department of general practice.

Sir James Mackenzie graduated in medicine from Edinburgh University in 1878. While a general practitioner in Burnley he developed an international reputation for his work in clinical research, mainly in cardiology. After time in practice in London, he returned to Scotland and in 1919 established his Institute of Clinical Research in St Andrews, but he was in poor health and died in 1925 before it became properly established. In 1963, his daughter endowed a chair of medicine in relation to general practice in his memory, and Richard Scott became the first professor of general practice in the world. The trustees of the original dispensary donated the premises (now named Mackenzie House) and their remaining funds to the university, and in 1969 the Cowgate practice was amalgamated with the West Richmond Street practice, although the academic offices remained in the Cowgate.

In 1983, after two relocations, the academic offices and the NHS practice were brought together in Levinson House (made possible by generous help from Simon Levinson – a local businessman), next door but one to Mackenzie House. Since then, the adjoining property has been purchased (with help from Stuart Pharmaceuticals), and the two buildings joined and extended. More recently the department has acquired further space in the old medical school buildings at Teviot Place to accommodate its expanding academic activity. Times move on, and as is happening in most medical schools, the academic disciplines of public health and general practice have again been united, and each recreated as units within a new joint department.

The development of this enterprise over sixty years has relied on the effort, goodwill and support of many people – too many to mention individually. Donald MacLean was Richard Scott's anchor in the original NHS practice, providing a hugely important role as both clinician and academic from 1953 until his retirement in 1990. Jane Paterson (the almoner in the practice) became – along with Mike Porter and Eileen Ineson (from the Manchester department) – one of the three founder members of AUTGP who were not medically qualified. The clinical load in the practice has consistently limited the opportunities for staff to develop their own research interests, and amongst many former staff from the early years of the department are David Morrell and Luke Zander (founder members of the St Thomas's department in London), Chris Donovan (who led developments at the Royal Free) and John Walker (who went on to establish the department in Newcastle). John Bain (later professor in Southampton and then in Dundee) was a trainee in the department, as was Bill Shannon who became professor of general practice at the Royal College of Surgeons in Ireland in Dublin. Those who stayed included Ian Stevenson (the first treasurer of AUTGP), whose early work on appointments systems was carried out in his own practice in Ayrshire, and Donald Thomson, who is now the faculty's admissions director.

Many local general practices took students on attachment on a voluntary basis (sixty are now regularly involved) before proper payment became available through ACT monies in the early 1990s. Over the years, they have provided a highly rated experience for generations of medical students, who now receive their introductory clinical teaching in general practice as well as two full-time attachments in their senior years – overall some 15 per cent of the clinical course.

Developing relevant research was always a major raison d'être of the department, but – especially in the early years – was difficult to achieve alongside the substantial clinical responsibilities of a busy inner-city practice. The department contributed usefully to early descriptive studies mapping the daily work of general practice, and took a decisive step forward when John Howie (professor from 1980–2000) and Mike Porter brought social and medical science thinking together to develop a long-term programme of researches on the determinants of good quality care at general practice consultations, with emphasis on the core values of patient-centredness.

The availability of ACT money from 1992 onwards allowed the department to recruit new staff to support the department's clinical work, to fund the network of supporting practices properly, and to create a proper research infrastructure – consisting mainly of social scientists. These included Sally Wyke (the first director of the Scottish School of Primary Care) and Margaret Maxwell, who are now professors at the University of Stirling, David Heaney, now with the Centre for Rural Health (associated with the University of Aberdeen), and Jane Hopton, now in management with Lothian Health. This team helped the department to achieve star ratings in the 1992 and 1996 RAEs. In addition, John Campbell is now a professor at the Peninsula Medical School, and four early research fellows are in chairs in Hull York (David Blaney), Christchurch (Les Toop), Dundee (Bruce Guthrie) and Canberra (Marjan Kljakovic), all helping fulfil the vision that Crew and Scott had embraced the better part of a half century previously.

Close working relationships with successive regional advisers (Alastair Donald, Graeme Buckley, Bill Patterson and David Blaney) and their teams, and regular meetings with them and officers of the LMC and College faculty, helped facilitate medical audit and research ethics activity in the 1980s, and contributed to the founding of the SSPC in the 1990s.

David Weller became professor in 2000, bringing a new research emphasis on cancer epidemiology and care, integrating well with strengths in the department of public health. The broad theme of whole-person medicine has been carried forward by the subsequent appointment of two professors with different but complementary skills in allergy, respiratory medicine and e-health (Aziz Sheik) and in primary palliative care (Scott Murray). The department that was the first to be created round a working NHS practice is now the only one in the UK left working with the same model – a model which relies on the availability of the same NHS support as applies in teaching hospitals to allow it to work successfully.

Dick Scott's legacy can be seen worldwide, although it has probably never been fully acknowledged publicly. His influence in advising on similar enterprises to his own – elsewhere in the UK, throughout Europe, and in Canada and Australasia in particular – was as important to the development of an academic base for the clinical discipline of general practice as was the substantial contribution he made to broadening the base of the Edinburgh medical school from 1947 until his retirement in 1979.

*John Howie*
*David Weller*

## Note

1. Thomson D.M., 'General Practice and the Edinburgh Medical School: 200 years of teaching, care and research', *JRCGP*, 34, 1984: 9–12.

# Chapter 4

# The University of Glasgow

## Background

The origins of the department in Glasgow lay partly in community medicine and partly in the concerns of the SHHD to develop health centres. Community medicine was represented in Glasgow by the department of epidemiology and preventive medicine based at Ruchill Hospital. Its head, Professor Tom Anderson, was a moving spirit in promoting the concept of a health centre combining clinical care with teaching medicine in the community. As early as 1964, a working party from the west of Scotland faculty of the College of General Practitioners recommended setting up a department of general practice under the chair of medicine.

In 1971, the Woodside Health Centre was opened with accommodation for eight practices covering about 40,000 patients. The records were combined in one office with an open plan reception area, treatment room and facilities for outpatient clinics, physiotherapy and X-rays. The centre also offered community dentistry and a wing for local authority clinics. Including facilities for teaching and research, Woodside paved the way for the development of academic general practice in Glasgow.

In 1972, Hamish Barber was appointed senior lecturer in primary medical care. The post was a joint one between the departments of medicine and of epidemiology and preventive medicine. It was funded by the Nuffield Provincial Hospitals Trust before becoming a university funded post. Barber's task was not easy as he had to work with two heads of departments with different interests: Gordon Stewart, professor of community medicine, and Edward McGirr, professor of medicine. In order to persuade the faculty that general practice should be allocated curriculum time, Barber had to demonstrate that after a trial period of teaching, students who had been through a general practice module out-scored a control group who had not.

## The department

In 1974, the department was established with the appointment of Hamish Barber to the Norie Miller chair of general practice funded by the General Accident Insurance Group. David Hannay was appointed senior lecturer, and Stuart Murray joined the staff as a research fellow (funded by the Nuffield Foundation) before becoming a senior lecturer. Subsequently John MacKay was appointed as a part-time tutor and later Joyce Watson became a research fellow.

The new department was housed in three rooms on the first floor of the Woodside Health Centre, between a seminar room and community dentistry. Eventually more accommodation was acquired in the attached local authority clinic. The department was practice-linked rather than practice-based, and the three full-time academic staff were attached to practices in the health centre as honorary principals with a commitment to three half days of service work a week.

In the 1980s, David Hannay became professor of general practice in Sheffield, and Stuart Murray was appointed postgraduate adviser to the west of Scotland. During this time Frank Sullivan, Jill Morrison and Tim Usherwood joined the department with SHHD fellowships. All three went on to hold chairs in general practice in, respectively, Dundee, Glasgow and Sydney. Jill Morrison became head of the undergraduate medical school, one of the first general practitioners to do so.

In 1994, Hamish Barber was succeeded by Graham Watt, and the department moved from Woodside to more spacious accommodation at Lancaster Crescent, and then to Horselethill Road. Una Macleod joined the department as the UK's first clinical research fellow in primary care oncology, funded by Cancer Research UK, before moving to a chair at Hull York University. Lisa Schwartz and Jane Macnaughton gained chairs in health care ethics at McMaster and in medical humanities at Durham. Phil Cotton and Peter Barton developed international profiles in medical education.

## Undergraduate teaching

Prior to 1972, medical students were offered only a week's voluntary general practice attachment during the fifth year, organised by Willie Fulton, who also gave two lectures. Later there was an opportunity for an elective in general practice. When Hamish Barber was appointed, a new five-year curriculum was being introduced to replace the existing six-year course. However, at the request of final-year students in the old course, a voluntary attachment to general practice was arranged and evaluated.

Hamish Barber's priority was to establish teaching in the new curriculum. At first, voluntary sessions in the old curriculum became compulsory in the new curriculum, with an emphasis on seeing patients in their own homes. A scheme was also introduced with the department of child health for students to visit disabled children at home.

Teaching in general practice evolved so that there was a general practice component in each of the clinical years with an emphasis on teaching medicine in the community, but without an examination in general practice. In the third year, students were released from hospital clinics to see the early presentation of illness in general practice, with an option to use videotape recordings for interviewing skills. There was also a half-day release to assess elderly patients at home. In the fourth year, students had twelve half days in general practice on the management of chronic illness, with opportunities for computer assisted learning. They were also taken to see patients with infectious diseases at home.

Organising teaching was a considerable task involving fifty to 100 general practice tutors, who received little recompense. In addition, staff did joint teaching in the third integrated year, including at the bedside in hospitals. In the third and fourth year there were student electives, involving thirty practices from the Borders to the Western Isles. One student project from these was published. All teaching initiatives were evaluated, and some were discontinued, such as an intercalated BSc course due to time constraints, and teaching interviewing skills due to curriculum changes. This teaching did not become a formal part of the curriculum until 1983, in a second year course on environment, behaviour and health.

In 1992, Jill Morrison led the introduction of a four-week attachment in general practice for final-year students, including problem-based learning and an audit project. The development of this course set precedents for educational planning which influenced the expansion of general practice contributions to the course during the next decade.

The increasing availability of NHS funds for undergraduate teaching and the opportunities offered by the new Glasgow curriculum resulted in new courses being developed and teams of general practice tutors being recruited. A novel feature of the new course was its provision of vocational studies, involving a general practice tutor meeting the same group of students once a week during the first and second years to address a range of professional issues. Overall, general-practice-based teaching accounted for about 16 per cent of the clinical course.

## Postgraduate teaching

Although departments of general practice had no responsibility for postgraduate training, when Stuart Murray became an associate adviser in general practice, the department had a formal involvement with vocational training. In 1972, the department of epidemiology and preventive medicine ran a two-month course on community medicine for vocational trainees which was taken over by the department and by 1977 was called 'The health of the community'. As well as specific topics there was also computer assisted learning and sessions on interviewing skills using videotape feedback with social workers trained as simulated patients.

In 1978 the department initiated a three-month course on 'Teaching methods in general practice' for small groups of teachers and trainers. In 1980, the four departments of general practice in Scotland were involved in an 'Extended course in general practice' for general practice trainers over the course of a year. That same year, the department also began contributing to the nursing degree course.

In 1982, the first MSc in general practice in the UK was started by the Glasgow department. The course was for one year full-time, or longer part-time. In its first year there were five general practitioners from the UK and two from Nigeria. The course covered research, educational methods, interviewing and counselling skills, and clinical areas, with a research project accounting for 50 per cent of the examination. Continuation of the Masters course depended on funding for prolonged study leave. In 2000, a successful multidisciplinary Masters programme in primary care was introduced, co-ordinated by Sandra McGregor.

The Higher Professional Fellowship Scheme in general practice, introduced by NHS Education in Scotland (NES), remains the most significant Scottish initiative in supporting careers in academic general practice, having produced five current members of staff, including Professor Stewart Mercer, whose CARE (Consultation and Relational Empathy) measure for assessing patient reports of doctor empathy has been translated into many languages.

## Research and publications

Evaluation of the developments in teaching resulted in a number of papers, such as Stuart Murray's work with computer assisted learning which led to a PhD, and David Hannay's work on teaching at McMaster which led to an MD. Indeed the principles of self-directed problem-based learning and continuous assessment permeated the teaching of general practice and influenced subsequent revisions of the medical curriculum in Glasgow. Some papers arising from David Hannay's research into illness behaviour were published as *The Symptom Iceberg* in 1979. John Goldie, an Easterhouse general practitioner, obtained his MD based on student responses to ethical dilemmas.

Other publications reflected Hamish Barber's pioneering work on health visitor programmes of prevention for children and care of the elderly. At one time, half the general practices in Scotland were using his Woodside child health record. In 1975, Hamish Barber produced a textbook entitled *General Practice Medicine*, with contributions from members of the department and others. In order to stimulate research by general practitioners he also built a portfolio of clinical trials funded by pharmaceutical companies, which supported part-time research appointments for service general practitioners. In 1977, the department organised the annual meeting of the then AUTGP. In the event, there were barely enough papers to fill the two-day event. However, during the first five years of the Glasgow department, some fifty papers were published with one of the three full-time members of the department as first-named author.

More recently, Phil Wilson led the Babycheck evaluation in local practices, paving the way for Westnet, which became the west of Scotland centre of the Scottish PCRN. Stuart Wood ran the Stepdown study of inhaled corticosteroids in asthma, recruiting the largest ever number of local practices without pharmaceutical funding. Jill Morrison's study of infertility guidelines was the first to randomise all Glasgow practices in a clinical trial. Kate O'Donnell led a series of national evaluations, including NHS 24, Keep Well and the new GMS contract, before gaining a personal chair. Graham Watt and Mark Upton led the MIDSPAN Family Study, adding over 2,300 adult offspring to the original Renfrew and Paisley Study, leading to publications on family-based topics. Graham Watt also led studies on the impact of deprivation on general practice, culminating in 'General Practitioners at the Deep End' initiative, involving the 100 most deprived practices in Scotland.

## Conclusions

The first ten years of the department were an exciting time, when those involved were at the forefront of developing general practice as an academic discipline. This foundation was built upon to provide an integrated programme of teaching, research and professional development in a department with a convivial, collegiate environment.

*David Hannay*
*Graham Watt*

# Chapter 5

# The Cardiff University School of Medicine

A medical school associated with Archie Cochrane's MRC epidemiology research unit and Professor C.R. Lowe's multidisciplinary university department of social and occupational medicine was ideally placed to develop academic general practice as an interface between biomedicine and community medicine. In 1968, Robert Harvard Davis, an Oxford graduate and general practitioner in Cardiff, was appointed to Professor Lowe's department to establish an academic unit of general practice with teaching and research responsibilities. He established a presence in the department of social and occupational medicine and then negotiated with Cardiff City Council to co-fund the building of an academic health centre on a new housing estate (Llanedeyrn) on the outskirts of Cardiff. The Welsh National School of Medicine (part of the University of Wales) supported the development and backed Harvard Davis as he raised charitable money and secured NHS cooperation in the establishment of a model NHS general practice that served the population of the Llanedeyrn area and provided clinical teaching for medical students. Facilities for general practitioners, nurses, health visitors, social workers, physiotherapy and pharmacy were included in the building plans: a model for teamwork.

A temporary building provided accommodation for the rapidly growing practice until 1971 when Llanedeyrn Health Centre opened. It was staffed by a combination of young academic general practitioners who worked in the practice and for the university, together with some older practitioners who worked part-time in their own practices and part-time in the academic unit at Llanedeyrn. Most of the funding for these posts came from NHS sources during the 1970s, with minimal university funding. Three quasi-independent 'clinical firms' consisting of senior lecturer, lecturer and registrar were established so that patients could develop continuity of care with their doctor of choice, but within a larger group practice framework. Even the ancillary staff were streamed in this way. Modern A4-sized medical records replaced the old Lloyd George envelopes and off-line computers at the university captured data for clinical research purposes, long before PCs arrived. A busy and forward-looking multidisciplinary health centre was fully functional by the time Prince Charles the Prince of Wales conducted the official opening of the building in 1972. He was impressed by early clinical audit activity.

Any introduction to the development of academic general practice in Wales would be incomplete without recognition of the pioneering work and publications of Julian Tudor Hart and W.O. Williams who ran the RCGP epidemic observation unit from 1973. Both men, working from their own practices, made major contributions to the international development of the discipline of general practice and to primary health care. Another pioneer was Derek Llewellyn, the first regional adviser for Wales: he led the development of vocational training for general practitioners in Wales during the 1970s.

Robert Harvard Davis travelled all over Wales with Derek Llewellyn to establish a range of undergraduate and postgraduate teaching and training practices. Back in Cardiff he was supported by his first lecturer (Brian Wallace), who helped mastermind the first clinical teaching programmes. Nigel Stott came to lead on clinical research developments, often in collaboration with the department of social and occupational medicine, soon to become a division of community medicine embracing epidemiology, public health, medical statistics, general practice and health visiting.

During the later 1970s most of these academic components became more autonomous. General practice was no exception; autonomy came early under a director (Robert Harvard Davis) and full professorial separation eventually occurred. The fragmented community medicine did not inhibit research collaboration between academic components but the geographic separation made communication less easy and a very heavy clinical workload also took its toll on academics.

By the end of the 1970s academic general practice was forging ahead in terms of student and academic acclaim. A social anthropologist, Roisin Pill, joined the staff as a research fellow and publication of original work on teaching and research fronts was commonplace. Funding was a major headache because the university expected the NHS earnings of the practice to pay for most academic costs. Furthermore the clinical academics on university salary scales were severely disadvantaged in comparison with their full-time service colleagues yet they carried heavy clinical responsibility and suffered the growing university pressure to win research grants for the kudos, funding and publications that followed. This was a national problem with an impact on recruitment and retention of staff.

When Robert Harvard Davis retired in 1986 he left a thriving multi-disciplinary department of general practice based on an expanded Llanedeyrn Health Centre and an NHS general practice. The latter was the responsibility of the head of department in collaboration with senior clinical staff, all of whom worked at Llanedeyrn and were in contract with both the university and the NHS. Undergraduate students were taught at the centre as well as in a network of teaching practices throughout the Principality. Close cooperation over postgraduate training was always fostered.

Nigel Stott succeeded Robert Harvard Davis as professor and head of department. He came into post as government policy began to question the old monopolies in health care provision and to force competition on a service that was not accustomed to competitive tendering or aggressive budget management. The 'internal market' had been born and with it came the certainty that clinical academics would not be allowed the service flexibility and freedoms that had enabled the development of academic general practice within a relatively relaxed NHS funding stream. There seemed no alternative other than to have an external review by management consultants from the King's Fund; this was followed by a negotiation for a new contracted funding stream from the NHS and the division of clinical and academic functions with each separately funded. The university was persuaded that there had to be an end to the casual reliance on NHS funding for a successful academic department of general practice. A 'Service Increment for Teaching' (SIFT) was negotiated with the Welsh Office while planning continued for the NHS practice to be ceded to a full-time lead partner, with more normal partnership arrangements.

Departmental initiatives in teaching, service and research into palliative care were now blossoming and a successful MPhil and Doctoral programme was developed. These busy years were also associated with the growth of much greater accountability in the national research funding arena. In addition a huge expansion of the role of general practice/primary care in undergraduate education was kindled by the GMC. Systematic teaching quality assessments across the whole university sector were launched.

During the 1990s the department was highly rated on each national teaching quality assessment. In addition the returned staff were rated five on successive RAEs, clear indications of international competitiveness.

Stott and Harvard Davies were responsible for an internationally important paper that outlined a framework for encouraging clinicians to explore and use the 'exceptional potential in each primary care consultation'.[1] The research output was extensive and included Stott and Pill's series of studies on the views of working-class women on health promotion, which continue to inform thinking about health promotion to this day. Other staff who have produced significant research findings include Paul Kinnersley, Glyn Elwyn, Adrian Edwards, Clare Wilkinson, Stephen Rollnick, Kerry Hood, Chris Butler and Tom O'Dowd, many of whom have gone on to have personal chairs of their own.

Nigel Stott retired in 2000, the year the University of Wales College of Medicine merged with Cardiff University, and Chris Butler became head of the newly combined department of primary care and public health at Cardiff University.

*Nigel Stott*
*Chris Butler*

## Note

1. Stott N.C.H. and Davis R.H., 'The exceptional potential in each primary care consultation', *JRCGP*, 29, 1979: 201–5.

# Chapter 6

# Academic General Practice in Ireland

Two of the original twenty-nine departments of general practice which came to constitute the AUTGP were based in Ireland, one at Queen's University Belfast (QUB) and the other at Trinity College Dublin (TCD). Over the years, cross-border collaboration led to the institution of the Association of University Departments of General Practice in Ireland (AUDGPI) in 1997. The 'Ireland story' presented in this chapter describes the early days of each department separately, followed by some reflections on how the partnership between them has now been formalised.

## Queen's University Belfast

In 1958, Professor John Pemberton, epidemiologist and founder of public health medicine, was appointed to the chair of social and preventive medicine at QUB. He spent time every summer as a locum with Will Pickles in the Yorkshire Dales, before retiring in 1976. He believed that medical students should be taught in general practice to see the influence of psychosocial factors on clinical decision-making and observe disease at an early stage as well as the management of chronic illness. In the early 1960s he arranged for students to visit general practices.

Pemberton wanted to create a teaching health centre close to the medical school, and was supported in this by the then Dean Sir John Henry Biggart. George Irwin was appointed to a part-time lectureship within Pemberton's department to develop teaching and research in primary care, laying the foundations for a future chair in general practice. In 1968, the General Health Services Board Northern Ireland offered £59,000 to the university to establish the chair, and more funding came from other sources.

In 1971 George Irwin was appointed foundation professor, and the department became the fifth to be created in the UK and the first in Ireland. It started life in cramped academic accommodation at the Royal Victoria Hospital, Belfast, with Irwin retaining his principalship in the practice he had helped to create in 1952. Funding was provided almost entirely from outside sources. A lectureship and one clerical post were made available. Pemberton's belief in the importance of a strong department of general practice was reflected in his willingness to give half his curriculum time to the new department.

On 1 April 1979 a new academic career structure in general practice in Northern Ireland was implemented. Dunluce Health Centre, situated adjacent to the Belfast City Hospital, was planned as a purpose-built teaching health centre, and opened its doors to patients on 1 January 1980. It housed four NHS general practice partnerships. The medical academic staff of the department of general practice were integrated part-time into these practices to maintain clinical experience and to promote teaching and research in primary care. The department moved into the fourth floor and was equipped with closed-circuit television and two-way mirror facilities in the consulting rooms.

The department is now involved in teaching in the first, second, fourth and final undergraduate years, has an extensive research programme and provides a range of postgraduate courses for general practitioners. By the time Professor Irwin retired in 1990, a well-balanced and respected department had been created with much enhanced funding. His successor Phillip Reilly continued the work of strengthening clinical, teaching and research facilities associated with the department. The chair has been vacant since Professor Reilly's retirement in August 2009.

*George Irwin*
*Philip Reilly*

## National University of Ireland, Galway

Andrew Murphy was appointed to the foundation chair in general practice at NUI Galway in 1997. The department was initially supported by four local health authorities which made agreement problematical. In 1999 a formal funding concordat was reached with the North Western and Western Health Boards and progress became easier. Today the department has a second full chair in primary care (Peter Cantillon), a senior lectureship (Liam Glynn), three lectureships (Mary Byrne, Maureen Kelly and Anne MacFarlane), a university teacher (Barry O'Donovan) and, in collaboration with the Irish College of General

Practitioners (ICGP), a senior registrar (Kim Kavanagh). Peter Cantillon took over as head of department in 2009.

University-linked practices have been developed for clinical staff at Turloughmore, the Claddagh and Ballyvaughan together with a network of almost 100 teaching practices along the western seaboard. Most of these practices are also part of an embryonic research network (http://westren.nuigalway.ie/index.html).

The department now has significant undergraduate teaching responsibilities in years one and four of the medical curriculum. Much emphasis was placed on developing postgraduate teaching and since 2001 a programme of higher Diploma, Masters and PhD in primary care has been available. In 2005, Peter Cantillon developed a programme for the Diploma and Masters in clinical education. Both these programmes now attract students on a national basis.

Research is focused on the themes of chronic conditions and multimorbidity, user involvement and medical education. The department, in conjunction with those at Trinity and Queen's, led the largest non-pharmaceutical trial conducted in Ireland – the SPHERE study (http://www.spherestudy.com).

The department has contributed to national policy-making through Andrew Murphy's involvement on the National Cardiovascular Strategy Advisory Group (2003–2007) and the Expert Group on Resource Allocation and Financing in the Health Sector (2009–2010). Peter Cantillon has been involved in developing the educational and dissemination strategies for the National Cancer Control Programme (2009).

*Andrew Murphy*

## Royal College of Surgeons in Ireland

In 1986 the Royal College of Surgeons in Ireland (RCSI) was the first of the medical schools in the Republic of Ireland to establish a chair in general practice. Bill Shannon, a Cork general practitioner and director of the Cork vocational training scheme, took up the foundation chair on 1 July 1987. One historically important condition negotiated by Bill was that the salary would have to equal that of the current professors of medicine and surgery, as the initial offer fell well below that of the other clinical professors. This significantly benefited future professors of general practice in the other Irish medical schools.

Bill recruited a large number of general practitioners to support his endeavours. He based his curriculum model, strongly emphasising communication and consultation skills, on those at Queen's University

Belfast and at the University of Edinburgh. In 1988 Gerard Bury was appointed as the first lecturer in general practice. In 1991 he went on to become the first professor of general practice at University College Dublin.

Tom Fahey was appointed professor in 2006, moving from a chair in Dundee. The department is now part of a larger division of population health sciences that includes epidemiology and public health as well as health psychology. The department has a network of more than seventy general practice tutors who provide clinical placements for over 300 students as part of their Early Patient Contact course in year two, and for over 250 students having their main general practice attachment in year four. Content is delivered via the Virtual Learning Environment, and assessment is moving towards combined assessment with other clinical disciplines such as medicine and surgery. The general practice undergraduate programme has a strong emphasis on evidence-based medicine and medical professionalism.

The research programme centres on the HRB Centre for Primary Care Research, a joint initiative led by RCSI and supported by academic colleagues in TCD and QUB (http://www.hrbcentreprimarycare.ie). This national programme of research is based on a collaborative approach with several academic departments contributing to the work, which includes medicines management in vulnerable groups (elderly, pregnant women, children and drug users) as well as an international register of clinical prediction that aims to identify, classify and combine Clinical Prediction Rules relevant to clinical practice in primary care. The register will be disseminated via the Cochrane Primary Health Care Field (http://www.cochraneprimarycare.org). Subsequently, we have become partners in an EU FP7 programme that is assessing patient safety with Information and Communication Technologies (TRANSFoRm). Lastly, the department contributes to the national HRB PhD scholars programme, and is supervising a cohort of young graduates from diverse health-related and health policy backgrounds.

*Bill Shannon*
*Tom Fahey*

## Trinity College Dublin

Jerry Jessop was professor of social medicine at Trinity College Dublin until 1973 when James McCormick, a general practitioner in Bray, took over, remaining in post until 1991. The title of the chair was changed to community health in 1977 to reflect wider changes. James put general practice firmly on the political and educational agenda in Ireland and set in train events which led to the establishment of the chair of general practice on his retirement, to which Tom O'Dowd was appointed in 1993. The department has always had a strong social medicine tradition which has allowed both primary care and public health to flourish and play a role in the national life. James was an internationally respected scholar, perhaps best remembered for his partnership with Petr Skrabanek and their iconoclastic views and writings on screening and about the epidemiology of cardiovascular disease.

Trinity, through the Mercer's Foundation, supported the development of a modern health centre in a deprived area in west Dublin, and the department takes part in the traditional final medical long case examinations. In 2004 undergraduate and postgraduate general practice united with the integration of the Trinity/Health Services Executive general practice training scheme into the department. This has allowed joint staff appointments, the involvement of general practice registrars in research, and access to well resourced practices for undergraduate teaching. The expansion of undergraduate general practice teaching now requires over 100 general practitioners, the department teaching in four out of the five undergraduate years.

The major research themes of the department are chronic disease, and the use of drugs and alcohol, and Tom O'Dowd is on the study team of 'Growing Up in Ireland', the national longitudinal study of 18,500 children.

In 2009, Joe Barry was appointed professor of population health medicine.

*Tom O'Dowd*

## University College Cork

In 1982 George Irwin was invited to Cork to speak on the role of general practice in the curriculum of his medical school at QUB. His message, to an audience of mainly University College Cork (UCC) medical school dons, could be summed up in one sentence: 'It is time for medical schools such as UCC to set up a department of general practice so that Cork graduates can receive a more balanced education and training in both hospital and community-based clinical settings.' Cork was not ready for George's clear message. Nor was it prepared to act when the same advice was given by John Howie from the University of Edinburgh, who wrote a succinct report to the then Dean of the medical school, Professor Robert Daly, following his two visits in 1983 and 1984. In contrast, the

Cork postgraduate vocational training scheme in general practice based at UCC went from strength to strength in the 1980s under the direction of Cork general practitioner Bill Shannon. Moves to set up a department of general practice began in 1989 when Tom O'Dowd was offered the new chair of general practice. It was to be partly funded from practice-generated income. This generated opposition among local general practitioners and, despite protracted negotiation, contributed to a parting of the ways between O'Dowd and UCC. Lessons were learned and in 1997 Colin Bradley was successfully appointed to the foundation chair in general practice.

Students now visit practices in year two once a month for basic skills training and have three-week attachments in year three and four weeks in year five. General practice now features in the final clinical examination. There are teaching links with over 100 practices in the Munster area and a research project has compared hospital and general practice teaching. The department supports the Diabetes Interest Group now comprising twenty-eight practices which have also provided a platform for research. Through involvement in the Strategy for Antimicrobial Resistance in Ireland the department has developed research into strategies to improve prescribing. The department has also collaborated with other departments, including economics and applied social studies and the school of pharmacy, in the areas of prescribing and medicines use.

*Bill Shannon*
*Colin Bradley*

## University College Dublin

In 1991, University College Dublin established its first chair in general practice with the appointment of Gerard Bury. UCD is Ireland's largest medical school, drawing students from all over Ireland and from abroad, particularly from Malaysia and North America. The importance of a primary care perspective to this audience was recognised early on, and the development of the department of general practice has been reflected in significant teaching roles for general practice in the four, five and six-year programmes available at UCD. The department was initially based at the Earlsfort Terrace home of the school of medicine, with a clinical base in the nearby inner city. With the opening of a major health sciences centre at Belfield, most early teaching has moved to the university campus and a major network of teaching general practices (currently almost 150) has been developed. The introduction of four-year graduate entry programmes has also been a significant driver in developing general practice sites for student placements starting in the first year.

A major theme of general practice at UCD has been the recruitment of general practitioners to academic life. The Coombe Healthcare Centre in Dublin's inner-city heartland is the shared clinical base for academic staff. It underpins the clinical, professional and psychosocial themes of the modules delivered by general practice. Professors Walter Cullen and Andrew Murphy were key members of staff moving to Limerick and Galway respectively. At the other end of the spectrum, the practice now hosts general practice interns – a learning enterprise for us all!

Research and development themes include emergency care, drugs misuse, infectious diseases, chronic disease management and medical education.

*Gerard Bury*

### University of Limerick

In Ireland, reforms in medical education policy (including increased student experience in primary care and the introduction of graduate entry programmes) were key to the establishment of Ireland's youngest medical school at Limerick University.

With a first student intake in 2007, our 'graduate entry' programme has benefited from the support of colleagues at other medical schools internationally (especially St George's in London) and in Ireland, and from primary care in Ireland's mid-west region. This year, fifty-eight students will complete an eighteen-week clinical module in general practice/ primary care, which is led by the foundation professor of general practice, Walter Cullen, and the school's director of education, Bill Shannon.

The school's strong primary care orientation is reflected in its research strategy, with mental health and substance-use disorders, hepatitis C, care of the elderly and multi-morbidity, and education in primary care among the active research themes. The first PhD studentship in primary care commenced in October 2010.

*Walter Cullen*

### Association of University Teachers of General Practice in Ireland (AUDGPI)

In the foreword of the 2002 Howie/O'Cuinneagain report on academic general practice in the Irish Republic, Michael Boland wrote: 'the creation of chairs and departments of general practice were amongst the most important aspirations of the founders of the Irish College of General Practitioners in 1984. Naively perhaps it was assumed that a professorial appointment would be accompanied by a critical mass of academic staff, a significant role in the curriculum, funding for teaching practices and a research agenda.'[1]

Curricular reform in Irish medical schools has been driven externally by the Irish Medical Council. The first general practitioner president of the Medical Council, Gerard Bury, made medical education reform a key platform for the Council. Tom O'Dowd was the first general practitioner chair of the Council's education committee between 1999 and 2004. Together they led detailed inspections of the medical schools and produced two key reports for a public audience concluding that medical education in Ireland needed urgent reform. The reports stated that medical education was unbalanced and underfunded and that international innovations in medical education were viewed with suspicion.[2] Public concern was such that the government established a commission to review medical education, including Professors Bury and O'Dowd among its membership.[3] The commission sought and received the views of the public and the medical profession and recommended increased funding for student places, introducing graduate entry (in parallel with traditional entry) programmes and an increased role for primary care. The government acted surprisingly quickly, providing increased funding which has led to new appointments, more student places, graduate entry and a new medical school at the University of Limerick.

The formal establishment of the AUDGPI in 1997 has provided a network and forum for academic departments on the island of Ireland to work together in teaching and research. The AUDGPI also provides an all-island rotating forum for the dissemination of research through an annual scientific meeting which regularly attracts up to 100 participants.

*Tom O'Dowd*

### Notes

1. Howie J. and O'Cuinneagain, F., *Realising the Potential: a report on the present position and future needs of departments of general practice in the medical schools of Ireland*, AUDGPI, 2002.
2. 'Review of Medical Schools in Ireland'. Reports to the public by the Medical Council, 2001 and 2003.
3. Working Group on Undergraduate Medical Education and Training, *Medical Education in Ireland: A New Direction (the 'Fottrell Report')*; http://www.dohc.ie/publications/fottrell (2006).

# Chapter 7

# The University of Birmingham

## 1974–1991

During the 1950s a number of Birmingham practices began to offer an informal experience of general practice to students in their elective period. Some offered contacts in the evenings or at weekends to students who requested this. The Birmingham LMC was active in encouraging such experiences. In 1966 the Midland faculty of the then College of General Practitioners began to explore the possibility of establishing a formal post in the medical school and Michael Drury, who had recently returned from a Nuffield Fellowship, was offered a part-time post as a lecturer in the department of social medicine by Professor Thomas McKeown. This enabled these elective attachments to be promoted more formally and with clear objectives and assessments.

These became sufficiently well taken up for the Dean, a neurosurgeon Professor Brodie Hughes, to agree that if outside money could be found for four years a part-time post with secretarial help would be established. Money was raised, principally thanks to the activities of two members of the faculty board, Micky Dale and Robin Steel, partly from a private donation and partly from a voluntary levy introduced by all the LMCs in the area. This enabled an appointment committee to be established in 1974 and Michael Drury was duly appointed Clarkson (named after the private donor) senior clinical tutor on a half-time basis. There was considerable discussion about where this post should be based. Both social medicine and clinical medicine were possibilities, but eventually clinical medicine under Professor 'Bill' Hoffenberg was chosen on the grounds that the task of the general practitioner was primarily that of a personal doctor and his community role, whilst important, was secondary.

It seemed that the best point in the curriculum to make a start was in the final-year four-month period of medical clerking in the department of medicine, and this was strongly supported by all the members of the department. Students were briefed for one morning in the medical school and then went in groups of four to one of four 'inner ring' practices in Birmingham. These were all large and well-known practices (three of them with close links to the College): Robin Pinsent and Laurie Pike in the north of Birmingham; Donald Crombie and partners (which already housed the College's research unit) in the west; Ray Davis and partners (one of whom, Douglas Fleming, later headed up the research unit) in the south; and Mick Houghton and partners in the east. They were paid a tiny honorarium for a week of structured teaching. The students then went to an 'outer ring' of some forty practices on a one-to-one basis for a further week before returning for a half-day debriefing session. These outer practices were 'rewarded' with a book token donated by a pharmaceutical company. Many students lived-in with doctors and their families for this second week and attended all the practice activities and night house calls. Some lasting relationships were formed and some students even ended up joining the practice as a partner.

To broaden the experience of students it was decided to take general practice teaching into the other major disciplines, surgery, paediatrics and obstetrics. Sessions were established in other hospitals where consultants would invite a general practitioner to attend a ward round including one of his patients after which, accompanied by Michael Drury, discussion would include how admission might have been avoided and what aftercare might be supplied. These 'before and after' sessions were not easy to arrange, partly through time constraints and partly because of the diffidence of the general practitioners, although almost always they came away encouraged by how much they were able to contribute.

Next came the establishment of lecture sessions on the place of general practice in community care, out of which arose a number of elective programmes looking at aspects of this work. The teaching of clinical pharmacology was always important in Birmingham and, around 1980, Professor Owen Wade involved the new sub-department of general practice in this each week. Together we began some research into general practice prescribing and later contributed to phase three clinical trials. Amongst our publications was *Treatment*, a textbook of drug therapy edited jointly by Owen Wade, Michael Drury and Linda Beeley, a clinical lecturer in pharmacology. We also devised a classification of drugs later taken on by Professor Wade to the BNF (British National Formulary) when he became its editor.

In the late 1970s the then Vice-Chancellor, Lord Hunt, who had a medical background, was persuaded that proper funding was needed. Money was provided for one part-time senior lecturer and two full-time research lecturers together with formal, if not over-generous payment and recognition of the four university teaching practices. We had calculated with Bill Hoffenberg the sum needed to support the four teaching practices, but Lord Hunt thought this was the sum required for each practice so in the event we secured four times the amount we had expected! Robin Hull, a general practitioner from nearby Stratford upon Avon, had been teaching on a short-term commitment at the University of Chapel Hill in North Carolina where Michael Drury had met him. Robin was offered the senior lecturer post, and eventually David Morgan and Andrew Carson joined as lecturers.

We expanded further into the curriculum. We had been worried that the exposure of students to live patients came so late that pre-conceived attitudes were already formed, so we introduced, amid much anxiety from other departments, a programme of early exposure in the first year. Our teaching practices were asked to invite families to allow a student to become attached to them for a year. Families were to include a patient with chronic illness, or an expectant mother, or a disabled adult or child. There was some anxiety that students might be drawn into difficult areas, so monthly tutorials were held with each student and a final report assessed in the examination programme. Problems rarely occurred and many lasting relationships were established. Students became god-parents, visited people throughout their five-year course, and became family friends.

Teaching of communication skills was a particular interest of Robin Hull and with the aid of the university film and video unit a busy programme was started. This then moved first into teaching sessions involving student nurses and physiotherapists, where team ideas could be explored, and, later, into joint sessions involving mature general practitioners and consultants. A presentation was given by Michael Drury at the Royal College of Physicians 'recent advances in medicine' course in Regents Park, after which he was asked by a member of the audience to speak to the charitable board of a merchant bank. As a result, a large donation was made enabling the setting up of a unit for teaching communication skills and the employment of specialist staff and equipment. Subsequently this donation was repeated.

Robin Hull had in the meantime secured a part-time appointment to a hospice in the region and this helped us to expose students to care for terminally ill patients. Another area of activity was education for general practice staff. This was a desert prior to the 1960s. Full-time training courses for medical secretaries or receptionists were started locally in the mid-1960s and soon spread nationally, eventually involving over 160 colleges. In the 1970s attention was turned towards nursing in general practice. A research nurse, Barbara Stillwell, who later became a nurse adviser to the World Health Organisation, joined the department, and studies were done on both practice nurses and, later, on the role of the first 'nurse practitioner', as we titled her.

In 1980 Michael Drury was appointed to a personal chair in general practice and the department became independent. Professor Drury served on a number of outside bodies, including the GMC, the Committee on Safety of Medicine, the Prescription Pricing Authority, the Standing Committee on Post-Graduate Education, as well as various committees of the RCGP, of which he became president in 1985, and was knighted in 1989.

## 1991–2002

The chair of general practice was formally established in 1991 when Michael Drury retired. Richard Hobbs, a senior lecturer in the department, took office from 1992 maintaining three weekly sessions in general practice. Between then and 1995 the priority was to expand staff numbers. This was to allow expansion of community-based teaching to meet the GMC requirements for more community exposure and behavioural sciences teaching, and to develop a strategic departmental research portfolio to compete at a national level. Three senior lecturer posts were created from limited capacity building by the university and significant funding from the NHS via the tasked funding for general practice initiative from the Department of Health. However, though senior lecturers were recruited, it was apparent that the pool of applicants was limited and future expansion required a bottom-up approach to develop new academics quickly. This was especially needed for research posts and, utilising newly awarded grants, a wave of clinical research fellows were appointed (now well-established senior academics). Amongst them was the first academic registrar to be appointed to general practice in the UK, David Fitzmaurice, and two recent trainees, Brendan Delaney and Yvonne Carter. In parallel, we established a formal research training programme through a Masters in primary care. The intention of these initiatives was to replace the self-taught academic career structure (often with a period in full-time service practice) that had been a common entrance to academia with early training in research methods and higher degrees.

The mid-1990s were therefore dominated by expanding community-based teaching and investment in research capacity building. A huge growth in student exposure to medicine based in general practice was supported by SIFT funding. This teaching was based in relatively few practices to enable a programme of significant capital investment for dedicated practice accommodation for teaching (two dedicated student consulting rooms and a seminar room/library for each practice) and major training of NHS teaching staff. Our contribution to the medical undergraduate programme expanded from a family attachment scheme in year one and two weeks in year five to a day in every alternate week of the first four years and four weeks in year five, with practices hosting students every week. Student intake increased from 120 to 160 in 1995, then to 250, and then 290 (peaking by 2002 at 450). Despite this exponential growth of new teaching load, quality remained high and was praised by the national assessment team in the university's 1999 HEFC QAA visit, with special citations for our innovative and ambitious CBT programme, medical ethics, and our teaching on ethnicity issues and communication skills.

The growth in research capacity required a longer horizon. The NHS had determined that research funding needed to be spent more strategically on applied clinical research and academic training plus improving delivery by directly 'compensating' the clinical service for supporting and hosting studies. At Birmingham, we capitalised on the new 'Culyer' initiatives, on which Richard Hobbs was the primary care representative, that resulted in the NHS R&D programmes (which subsequently evolved into the NIHR) in the late 1990s.

At a more senior research level, the mid-1990s was a period of better defining our research programmes, all unashamedly clinically focused, and expanding our major 'laboratory' of a research practices network. The latter had been established in 1985, initially mainly supporting commercial pharmaceutical trials which brought us two essential ingredients – funding (to develop the infrastructure) and scientific rigour in trial design and the strict governance procedures linked to early-phase drug trials. The funding to support our cardiovascular, gastrointestinal and cancer teams was won in the new NHS R&D applied clinical research funding streams, including a specific cardiovascular diseases panel, and a one-off MRC primary care research programme. The pivotal year for research successes was 1999, with the cardiovascular team winning two substantial MRC grants to study atrial fibrillation management by anticoagulation in over-75s (BAFTA), and anticoagulation self-monitoring (SMART), plus a large HTA programme grant to support a study into atrial fibrillation screening (SAFE). The scale of this programme may be gauged by the seventeen full-time new research posts created to support the three trials in 2000 and the expansion of our MidReC network to over 125 practices. The cardiovascular and gastrointestinal teams were rewarded with two of the first NHS R&D career scientist awards (out of seven awarded nationally in 1999).

Having been assessed at the very disappointing level of 3b (the second lowest grade) in the RAE of 1996, the exponential growth of the departmental research programmes from the mid-1990s in terms of size and quality was rewarded by a top ranking five-star RAE grade in 2001, one of only four such awards in primary care that year. One final essential ingredient in our progression was the plan for new accommodation, finally completed and occupied in April 2002, which, for the first time since 1992, allowed all of the various teams in the department to be located in the same building.

*Michael Drury*
*Richard Hobbs*

Chapter 8

# The University of Bristol

The medical faculty of the University of Bristol was slow to accept that general practice has a role in teaching medical students and was the last of the pre-2000 medical schools in the UK to create an academic undergraduate post occupied by a general practitioner. The story behind this development is interesting and illustrates the way that tradition can be challenged and eventually altered.

In the early 1960s, Bristol's professor of public health and medical officer of health, Robert Wofinden, created a name for himself with the development of health centres. He saw this as a way of bringing together general practitioners, nurses, midwives and health visitors to improve the health of patients in various parts of the city. At the same time Michael Lennard, a relatively recent Bristol graduate, was working in general practice in Hartcliffe, a new estate in the south of the city, and was keen to introduce medical students to general practice. In 1963 Sandy Macara (later president of the BMA) was appointed lecturer within the small public health department and given the responsibility for running a four-week general practice clerkship. In 1965 the southwest faculty of the College of General Practitioners sent a memorandum of evidence to the medical curriculum review committee of the university stating 'we strongly urge the setting up of a department of general practice as a logical step in the development of undergraduate medical education'.

The general practice input within the public health teaching enthused the medical students and the medical student society asked Dr Macara to conduct a survey of medical student opinion about the need to have dedicated time in general practice. The results were very positive and were presented to the medical faculty only to be resisted with comments from many of the senior professors that 'we can't have general practitioners teaching our students heresies'. Eventually, in the mid-1970s, with support from child health and the geriatricians, a new six-week course for the final year was agreed, called 'medicine in the community'. This course was intended to 'introduce students to medicine in the community', not to teach as such! Two weeks of this was to take place in practices throughout the region with some time spent in city practices. Doctors who took the students in their practices were rewarded with a university title of 'teacher in general practice' enabling them to have access to the medical library and sports facilities.

Postgraduate teaching of general practice was reasonably well financed and supported. Michael Lennard was appointed as regional adviser in general practice in the early 1970s for the whole of the south-west and this job was subdivided a few years later. The university recognised Michael Lennard as postgraduate adviser in general practice for Gloucester, Avon and Somerset, and Denis Pereira Gray as postgraduate adviser for Devon and Cornwall in 1975. The course organisers who had been appointed in 1975 were called 'recognised teachers in general practice' by the university in the same year. They ran the weekly half-day courses for aspiring general practitioners and organised the new vocational training courses throughout the region. These courses in the south-west were very popular and Exeter, in particular, developed considerable expertise in educational method and created a thriving postgraduate department of general practice under the leadership of Pereira Gray.

Having a well-organised postgraduate practice network was of great help in organising student placements throughout the region. However the faculty remained resistant to developing an academic presence in the medical school and missed at least one opportunity of obtaining central government funding for such a development. John Howie was appointed as the RCGP Jephcott visiting professor in 1979–1980 and his report to the university outlined the way to develop an independent department of general practice. A university working party report on how this new department could be developed had its proposals rejected and again the need for such a department was questioned.

One key development that eventually forced a change was the decision of general practitioners and consultants within the postgraduate education department in the south-west in 1985 to set up a charitable trust to raise money, primarily from general practices in the south-west, to support departments of general practice in the Universities of Bristol and Exeter. The Trust's target was £250,000 as a pump priming effort to stimulate major authorities in the region to fund the two departments – to start a department in Bristol and to permanently secure the one in Exeter. This had the almost immediate effect of obtaining funds from the south-west region and the university was able to report in November

1985 that 'the way is now clear for the appointment of a full-time consultant senior lecturer in general practice for a period of five years and a three year appointment of a consultant senior lecturer once the first appointment has been made and the successful candidate is in post'.

In 1986 Michael Whitfield was appointed full-time senior lecturer in general practice within the department of public health medicine, with the university funding five sessions and a full-time secretary. David Jewell was appointed a year later as senior lecturer. New funding brought in Chris Watkins as a part-time senior lecturer, and Richard Baker (who later moved to a chair in Leicester) and Lindsay Smith as part-time research fellows. A full-time chair was eventually funded by the south-west RHA and the university appointed Debbie Sharp to the position in 1994.

The timing of this appointment coincided with the first edition of the 1993 GMC publication *Tomorrow's Doctors* and with a radical rethink of the medical undergraduate curriculum that resulted in a new emphasis on communication and consultation skills, both of which were very much the domain of general practice. Very quickly, under Debbie Sharp's leadership, general practice was to be found in each of the five years of the undergraduate curriculum. This was helped a great deal by the support of the then FHSA who believed strongly in the student presence in practices helping to raise standards.

The other major fortuitous activity was the development of the NHS R&D initiative which in the mid-1990s had several commissioned calls for research that spoke strongly to the academic general practice agenda and skill base. This, together with further funds to appoint two lecturers in general practice, marked the beginning of an extremely successful research unit, initially as part of the then department of social medicine and later as an autonomous division in the medical school. As the grants were obtained more staff were appointed, a sufficient critical mass developed, high quality papers began to be published and a virtuous circle began. In addition there was early success in obtaining research training fellowships for both clinical and non-clinical primary care researchers and Bristol began to develop a name for itself in academic general practice circles as a good place to be.

Attracting high quality staff like Chris Salisbury and Tom Fahey, both of whom went on to gain chairs, ensured that Bristol became a force to be reckoned with on the UK academic general practice scene. By 2000 the medical school had clearly recognised the value of academic general practice, appointing Debbie Sharp as head of the school of medicine.

*Michael Whitfield*
*Debbie Sharp*

# Chapter 9

# The University of Cambridge

Medicine has been studied in Cambridge since 1318, but it was not until the time of John Butterfield (Regius 1976–1987) and Keith Peters (Regius 1987–2005) that the foundation chairs of community medicine (1977) and general practice (1996) were established. Butterfield led the establishment of the school of clinical medicine (1976), and Peters the transformation of the school into a world leading centre for medical research.

The path to realising the academic aspirations of general practice led uphill. The combined efforts of postgraduate general practice educators, the RHA, Royal Colleges and local practitioners took twenty years to establish a chair of general practice.

In the 1970s the Royal Commission on Medical Education[1] strongly recommended including general practice in the clinical curriculum, recognising it as a specialty and proposing structured general practice postgraduate training and senior academic appointments for general practice undergraduate teachers. In East Anglia, regional and associate general practice advisers were appointed in the postgraduate Dean's office, providing the first formal links between general practice education, the RHA and the university.

Bernard Reiss (the first regional adviser from 1973–1976) and Ian Tait (associate), held these key link positions. Having previously introduced pre-clinical student visits to local general practices they pushed for clinical teaching appointments and in 1976 hoped for a general practice undergraduate teaching and research department. The university responded by creating the post of director of studies in general practice.

## The first general practice undergraduate academic appointment

Reiss was appointed the first director of studies (1976–1987). The potential opportunity for an integrated school of general practice in Cambridge, offered by his holding both posts, was not however realised. There were barriers to development. The general practice community felt unable to influence the attitudes of senior academics, and the priority to establish the research faculty of the clinical school prevailed. The university's undergraduate clinical teaching and research were centred largely in Addenbrooke's Hospital. General practice teaching practices were appointed but the general practice community felt the lack of a dedicated department. A small compensation was the transfer of the postgraduate Dean's office to the clinical school building in 1980, bringing the new regional adviser (Bob Berrington) alongside the director of studies – though the two systems remained administratively and financially independent.

## The early general practice undergraduate curriculum

The Cambridge clinical course was six months shorter than other courses. Fierce competition for teaching time existed between hospital departments, and consultants all felt that their specialty was insufficiently recognised. There was little enthusiasm for finding curriculum time for general practice. Despite these difficulties, Reiss established an introductory day in general practice, a two-week attachment in phase II and, when the course was extended, a two-week senior attachment in general practice.

## Developing research: the Fenland research group

Roy Acheson (foundation chair of community medicine) was keen to enable general practice research.[2] In 1980 Reiss and Acheson, recognising that general practice research was a necessary precursor to a future department of general practice, convened a meeting of local general practitioners to gauge interest in forming a research group. The foundation members, who saw themselves as potential academics, were Noreen Caine, Hugh King, Nigel Oswald, John Perry, Jeffrie Strang, Ian Wallace, Stewart Warrender and Tony White. The group met regularly over eighteen years, obtaining funding and publishing papers.

## The McWhinney Report: 1983

In 1983 Ian McWhinney, at Reiss's instigation, was appointed RCGP Jephcott visiting professor in Cambridge. He found resistance to the expansion of general practice teaching amongst faculty of medicine members linked to a view that the clinical school's purpose was 'to attract future scientists rather than practitioners', though the proportion of undergraduates intending a general practice career was similar to other medical schools. McWhinney set out powerful arguments for a general practice department.[3] No action followed.

## Further development of academic general practice: 1987–1997

Nigel Oswald and Martin Roland were partners in the same practice as Reiss. Oswald's chief interest was in teaching and learning, Roland's in research. When Reiss retired both were keen to make a contribution. They were appointed to share the four-session director of studies post.

Oswald developed a new parallel course in Cambridge known as the Cambridge Community-based Clinical Course (CCBCC).[4] It received GMC and clinical school approval for an intake of four students per year from 1993, and was based on a fifteen-month continuous clinical attachment in Oswald's practice. Students gained experience by following individual patients from community to hospital and back.

This innovation raised the profile of general practice academics in Cambridge. It contributed to a national shift of opinion and practice towards primary care learning for students, especially in the new medical schools. It led to constructive relations with both the Dean and Regius, and to positive interaction with the GMC. Oswald was appointed to the GMC with a role in quality assurance of basic medical education. The CCBCC became paradoxically both a jewel in the teaching crown of the clinical school and a barrier to the expansion of general practice undergraduate teaching for the generality of students at Cambridge. The closure of the CCBCC paved the way for wider developments in teaching in the community on both the traditional course based at the clinical school at Addenbrooke's and the planned graduate course at the West Suffolk Hospital.

Roland had trained as a general practitioner in Cambridge, and then worked with David Morrell in the department at St Thomas's Hospital, before returning to work as a general practice principal highly active in research. His interest in quality of care, especially across the primary secondary care interface, is apparent in his health services research (HSR) publications from that decade.

## Building a general practice group and establishing a foundation chair

In 1987 Keith Peters was appointed as Regius. Oswald and Roland met him immediately to explore his attitude to developing a general practice department. Although he recognised that there was a good case, it was clear that what other schools were doing was not of consequence. A general practice department was not then on his agenda. His explicit priority was the development of medical research which he felt to be at a primitive level in Cambridge. He felt that teaching could remain in the hands of the Dean. He did not deny the possibility of a department of general practice in due course, but would give no immediate active help.

In the early 1990s, a contribution towards funding a Cambridge chair arose through contacts between Bob Berrington and the RCGP. However, the clinical school and general board did not judge that the resource, its commercial source or the timing were appropriate. The RHA was also not forward in offering support to fill any gaps. The view was that general practice did not have a strong enough research base and that there were unlikely to be general practice academics of the stature to occupy a chair in Cambridge. In 1992, with developments in Cambridge seeming increasingly unlikely, Roland accepted the post of professor of general practice in Manchester.

Oswald was now appointed to a full-time university lectureship. Two other general practice appointments as part-time directors of studies were made (John Perry and Tony White), followed by others associated with the clinical school ethics and communication agendas. By then (1989) the group had been accommodated within the Institute of Public Health where Nick Day had succeeded Acheson as head of the department. Academic general practitioners were recognised to be contributing strongly to the clinical school. However, none of this brought full department status any nearer.

In establishing new chairs, the Regius sought to appoint people with a proven track record from other universities. Although general practice research had developed widely by this time, only a few people had top credentials. In 1989, while visiting Cambridge to examine an MD thesis, Ann Louise Kinmonth first met the Regius and asked why he had not established a chair in general practice. He said he planned to do so within the next five years, and asked if he might visit the Southampton department. After his visit the Regius set up an implementation group on the selection and appointment of a professor of general practice.

In 1992, the Regius asked Kinmonth to advise him on the establishment of the chair while using the occasion of their meetings to show interest in her own career. Kinmonth had just accepted the chair of primary medical care in Southampton and told the Regius she would be unable to move soon. Given the speed at which Cambridge moved to set up its own chair this did not seem to offer much impediment.

In 1995, before any formal advertisement, Kinmonth was invited to dine with the Regius at Christ's 'to meet a few people'. These turned out to be the senior academic staff of the department of community medicine who all seemed fairly unclear as to the context of the invitation. The Regius, however, seemed very happy and hosted a convivial evening. There is no doubt that the Regius' leadership was the decisive factor in the establishment of the university chair. His experience of the negotiations, funding and procedures within the university was crucial to its eventual decision.

## The foundation chair

The Board of Electors invited applications for the professorship of general practice in April 1996. The chair was to be placed within the department of community medicine and Kinmonth was invited to apply. Aware of the considerable opportunities for establishing an active general practice research group to complement the thriving general practice education group led by Oswald and the active HSR group led by Chris Todd, she saw a gap to be filled in translational research. There was little work at the interface between the population and the individual or in trials to establish cost-effective practice. In particular, the emerging understanding of the natural history of diabetes and its behavioural determinants and the new approaches to objective measurement of health-related behaviours, especially physical activity, offered the possibility of transforming the quality and scope of the work Kinmonth had begun in Southampton. There was also exceptional access to other relevant disciplines from anthropology to statistics.

In general the 'flat' nature of the departmental hierarchy, the enabling approach of Nick Day and his openness to delegation of budgetary and strategic authority were reassuring. Also important were the wholehearted support of the general practice community, the postgraduate deanery (director Arthur Hibble) and the local faculty of the RCGP (provost Bob Berrington); and the enthusiasm of the regional directors of NHS R&D, Richard Himsworth and Muir Gray. Kinmonth applied and was elected to the chair.

Following the election, the Regius asked Day to sound out the conditions under which Kinmonth might accept the appointment. Day and Kinmonth met at the Royal College of Physicians to discuss this. The case put forward was seen as excessive by Cambridge, but as necessary by someone who had experience of running a department of general practice. Kinmonth was invited back to the Regius' office to meet Peters and Day. The Regius explained that there was only sufficient funding for the chair and not for the support posts proposed. Kinmonth formally declined the post and left the meeting. At this point the Regius called on Himsworth to negotiate an acceptable support package with the RHA and on this occasion the Authority moved strongly to enable a general practice unit to be established with a portfolio of funding support.

In January 1997 the general practice and primary care research unit was established integrating the HSR group, the education group and the new research group, under the direction of the chair. There were some tensions; for example it became clear that the new general practice research group was intended to replace the existing HSR group, at least to some extent. In the event the potential difficulty was overcome and Chris Todd proved a generous and collaborative colleague during the years before he accepted a chair in Manchester. In 1998 Nigel Oswald accepted the post of professor in primary health care, jointly in the Universities of Newcastle and Teesside. Simon Griffin (Southampton) and John Benson (Cambridge) were soon recruited to build the research and teaching strands respectively and close links formed with the deanery under its new director of general practice postgraduate education, Arthur Hibble.

The unit developed an integrated teaching and research academic mission linked to service; the research focus was on the development and evaluation of cost-effective strategies for the prevention of chronic disease, and the translation of research evidence into practice. The teaching aimed to offer evidence-based education to the doctors of tomorrow in a primary care setting. The department changed its name to the department of public health and primary care in recognition of the new establishment. The unit was awarded a five-star rating in its first RAE.

## Postscript

By 2010 the unit comprised four professors (Ann Louise Kinmonth, general practice; Stephen Sutton, behavioural science; Jonathan Mant, primary care; and Martin Roland, HSR), two senior lecturers (John Benson, director of education and associate dean; and Simon Cohn, social anthropology), one new blood university lecturer elect Stephen Barclay, and three senior visiting fellows (Simon Griffin, assistant director MRC Epidemiology Unit; Jon Emery, professor of general practice Perth Western Australia; and Theresa Marteau, professor of health psychology King's College London). The unit hosts two NIHR clinical lecturers (Fiona Walter and Nahal Mavadatt) and, with the deanery, a thriving academic clinical fellowship programme. Its high quality contributions to medical research and teaching are now well recognised both in Cambridge and internationally, amply justifying the university's decision on its foundation and subsequent support.

*Bob Berrington*
*John Perry*
*Nigel Oswald*
*Martin Roland*
*John Benson*
*Ann Louise Kinmonth*

## Notes

1. The Royal Commission on Medical Education 1965–68, London, HMSO, 1968.
2. Strang J., Caine N. and Acheson R., 'Practice research: team care of elderly patients in general practice', *BMJ*, 286, 1984: 851–4.
3. McWhinney I.R., Jephcott Visiting Professorship, Cambridge University. Final Report on the Assessment of General Practice in the Medical School, 1983.
4. Oswald N., Alderson T. and Jones S., 'Evaluating primary care as a base for medical education: the report of the Cambridge Community-based Clinical Course', *Medical Education*, 35, 2001: 782–8.

# Chapter 10

# The University of Exeter

The University of Exeter established a department of general practice on 1 December 1973, just before a postgraduate university department of general practice was established in Denmark. This was the first post-graduate university department of general practice in the UK, modelled on the London postgraduate medical institutes. It was funded by the DHSS to develop vocational training for general practice. For almost a year, Denis Pereira Gray was alone with a half-time appointment as senior lecturer, the only academic general practice presence in the south-west region. Three more part-time senior lecturers, Keith Bolden, Michael Hall and Robert Jones, joined in November 1974, creating the team soon known as the 'gang of four'.

Exeter became a laboratory for vocational training with radical ideas tested and evaluated. *A System of Training for General Practice* (1977) became the best-selling of the RCGP's early Occasional Papers and was followed by three books: *Training for General Practice*, *A GP Training Handbook* and *Running a Course*.

Academic features of the Exeter vocational training scheme included an emphasis on three-year training, the use of interactive small-group learning with behavioural de-briefing, rigorous selection of trainers, protected time for trainees in the practices for research, and support for trainees publishing research findings. Between 1974 and 1995, Exeter general practice trainees and one pre-registration doctor had seventeen articles published in the international peer-reviewed literature. Amongst these were an early report of high blood alcohol levels in patients in accident departments, and the statistically based 'value for money index' in general practice training. Later, Wakeford reported that Devon and Cornwall had the highest pass rate for the MRCGP of any region in the UK.

In July 1975, the University of Bristol established a second regional advisership (Devon and Cornwall) for Pereira Gray (the first had been for Michael Lennard in Bristol).

The selection of trainers was conducted rigorously, the adviser visiting in person virtually every applicant, and an annual Devon and Cornwall trainers' course was established. Keith Bolden and Michael Hall soon became associate advisers.

The integration of a university department with the regional adviser also occurred at Guy's, but only in Exeter was it sustained for a quarter of a century, fusing research, postgraduate education and clinical standard setting. The *JRCGP*, now the *BJGP*, was edited for nine years in Exeter and departmental staff between them wrote or edited the first book on practice management, the first on practice nursing, a history of the RCGP,[1] and *Psychiatry and General Practice Today*. Several of these books and booklets went into further editions. The RCGP Occasional Papers were designed, edited and published in Exeter for twenty-one years, as well as the RCGP Members' Reference Book for fifteen years, and the Medical Annual for five years.

In April 1983, to cover the longest mileage in England, three regional advisers in general practice were appointed by the University of Bristol with Roddy Hughes leading Gloucester, Avon and Somerset, Keith Bolden looking after Devon and Cornwall, and Denis Pereira Gray having all-regional responsibility.

Several consultancies for the World Health Organisation (WHO) in Geneva and Europe led to the department of general practice being invited to host and chair a week-long international seminar in July 1983 on the future of the European medical schools. WHO also invited several European Deans and the CMO for Scotland. Opened by a government minister, protocol required that the WHO flag flew from the hospital!

In 1983, after a decade of support from the DH, the department chose to go self-financing, thus achieving the freedom to develop academically. The priorities it adopted were broader than for many university departments and included research, multi-professional development, standard setting, postgraduate education, and leadership. Meanwhile, the University of Bristol repeatedly refused to establish a department of general practice despite requests and deputations.

In 1985, six general practitioners, led by three from Exeter, and three consultants – including Lord Richardson, former president of the GMC, as chairman – launched the South West General Practice Trust, a new registered charity to support general practice within the universities of Exeter and Bristol. An appeal to every general practice in the region generated generous donations, many practices covenanting £500 a year for seven years. This stimulated the RHA to donate to the Trust almost a million pounds. The Trust invited the then two Vice-Chancellors to an event, presented cheques, and secured a university department at Bristol.

This Trust continues twenty-five years later, with capital of about two-thirds of a million pounds.

In 1986, the department launched an MSc in health care, the first multi-professional Masters of its kind in the UK. People mortgaged to attend and the course developed into one of the biggest in Britain. General practitioners and allied professionals were encouraged to obtain higher university degrees through this MSc. Several local general practitioners and health professionals were supervised to achieve research MPhils and MDs.

Multi-professional staff appointed included Rita Goble, an occupational therapist who obtained King's Fund support for the first British multi-professional postgraduate training programme for physiotherapists, occupational therapists and speech therapists. The first three PhDs in occupational therapy came from Exeter, including a future chief executive of a PCT.

In October 1986, the university established a personal chair in general practice, the first chair of general practice in the south-west region and the third medical chair in Devon and Cornwall. In 1987, a sudden vacancy in the RCGP led to the appointment of Pereira Gray as Chairman of Council, the first professor so elected. On the retirement of the first director of the Exeter University postgraduate medical school (PGMS), Pereira Gray was nominated by both the consultant staff of the hospital and the specialist academic staff. The university subsequently appointed him the second director (Dean) of the PGMS from 1 April 1987, becoming the only general practitioner in such a position. He served as director for ten years during which time the PGMS received the university's first Queen's Anniversary Award.

The research programmes with multiple publications were on vocational training, continuity of care, contraception/abortion, terminal care and the national pilot on putting the medical record onto a patient-held card. Several publications attracted over 150 citations; these were on vocational training,[2] why general practitioners do not follow evidence (Freeman and Sweeney),[3] symptom attribution in depressed patients,[4] and the association between continuity of care and trust in patients.[5]

Professional development in British general practice was greatly stimulated by the Fellowship by Assessment (FBA) programme of the RCGP. The department of general practice was centrally concerned in the drafting and leadership of this and two of the staff, Tony Lewis and Russell Steele, were amongst the first nine general practitioners in the UK to achieve it. Close partnership with the Tamar (Devon and Cornwall) faculty led to these two counties producing thirty-two FBAs, several of whom later undertook higher university degrees.

Multi-professional education developed with staff in occupational therapy and management being appointed. Intensive courses were offered especially in practice management, consulting skills, personality analysis and transactional analysis. The department was appointed the first Centre of Excellence in Practice Management by the Association of Practice Managers.

International relationships developed, especially with Hungary, Egypt and Turkey. Several Hungarian leaders were funded to attend the department's MSc. In 1996, led by Keith Bolden, the newly promoted Institute of General Practice was awarded a teaching contract by the Egyptian government to train Egyptian family physicians. At £1m, this was the largest contract the university had received.

A unit teaching leadership skills on a Masters' course and to post-graduate students needs to demonstrate leadership roles itself. In the 1990s, Michael Hall was elected to the chair of the board of trustees of Diabetes UK (the first general practitioner to chair a multi-million-pound national charity), the presidency of the Association of Practice Managers came to Keith Bolden, and Bob Jones founded a new charity for people with severe physical disabilities. Staff delivered twenty-one eponymous lectures, four overseas. Former Exeter students (Kieran Sweeney and Martin Marshall) won Harkness International Fellowships and others gained leadership positions including four university chairs and the chairmanship of the NHS Alliance. Staff later received three university honorary doctorates and a university fellowship.

The Exeter Institute was honoured by successive elections of its head to the chairmanships of the Council of the RCGP, the Conference of Academic Organisations of General Practice, the Joint Committee on Postgraduate Training for General Practice, to the presidency of the RCGP, and by the presidents of the Medical Royal Colleges in Great Britain and Ireland, as the first and only general practitioner, to the Chairmanship of the Academy of Medical Royal Colleges.

*Denis Pereira Gray*

(Pereira Gray was succeeded as director of the Exeter postgraduate medical school in 1997 by Professor John Tooke. Pereira Gray was knighted for services to quality assurance in general practice in 1999 and retired as director of general practice education for the south-west region in 2000 and as professor at the Institute of General Practice of the University of Exeter in 2001. Tooke led the bid for a new medical school which was established in 2000 – see Appendix 1 – with him as Dean. Specialty-based departments were closed. John Campbell was appointed to the foundation chair of general practice and primary care in 2002.)

## Notes

1. Pereira Gray D. (ed.), *Forty Years On: The Story of the First Forty Years of the Royal College of General Practitioners*, London, RCGP, 1992.
2. Pereira Gray D.J., *A System of Training for General Practice. Occasional Paper 4*, second edition, Exeter, RCGP, 1979.
3. Freeman A. and Sweeney K., 'Why general practitioners do not implement evidence: a qualitative study', *BMJ*, 323, 2001: 1100–14.
4. Kessler D., Lloyd K.R., Lewis G. and Pereira Gray D.J., 'Recognition of depression and anxiety in primary care', *BMJ*, 316, 1999: 436–40.
5. Mainous A.G., Baker R., Love M., Pereira Gray D.J. and Gill J.M., 'Continuity of care and trust in one's physician: evidence from primary care in the US and UK', *Family Medicine*, 33, 1, 2001: 22–7.

# Chapter 11

# The University of Leeds

## Beginnings

Undergraduate teaching in general practice started life in the University of Leeds on 1 July 1974 as a division within the department of community medicine and general practice. The department was headed by Professor Gerald Richards, whose clear preference was that, in terms of educational and research policy, the new unit should have a considerable measure of autonomy.

Though vigorously supported by the then Dean (Professor Derek Wood), the creation of such a unit was regarded with derision by a few of the influential senior faculty staff. Curricular time was, consequently, limited at first to a fortnight in the students' final year.

Financial issues also loomed large. Some four years earlier the UGC had ruled that NHS fees and allowances earned by practitioners appointed to such a unit should be assigned to the university. There was to be no 'service increment for teaching' (SIFT) such as applied to hospital-based teaching units.

## Preparation

John Wright was appointed head of the division six months in advance and this enabled the selection of sixteen part-time 'tutors in general practice' – local practitioners who would take students regularly into their practices and meet monthly to review problems and progress. This also allowed time to gain experience from visiting other units, both in the UK and in Toronto and at McMaster in Canada.

The academic unit was accommodated in three rooms in a disused wing of St James's Hospital, alongside the university's departments of surgery, gynaecology and anaesthetics (a valuable arrangement allowing continuing conversation with them). More spacious accommodation came later in the newly built clinical sciences building, with similar proximity to paediatrics and psychiatry.

In November 1974 Douglas Macadam was appointed as a second senior lecturer, and Ian Stanley joined as a third in 1980. Further support in the early stages was provided through Paul Freeling's appointment as RCGP Jephcott professor in 1978, his series of visits stimulating involvement and support across a wide variety of interested groups. Given the severely restricted initial resources, the division's first priority was education, with research secondary and dependent on 'soft' money.

## Educational aims

The first task was to clarify the distinction between training and education. Training aims to prepare the individual for the particular tasks of the graduate's chosen career. Its hallmark is thus particularity. In contrast, the Royal Commission described the aim of undergraduate education as being 'not the production of a qualified doctor, but an educated man who becomes qualified in the course of postgraduate training'.

To achieve this, the course aimed to help the student develop first, the necessary cognitive skills (including observation, communication, hypothesis-formation, analysis of data); second, appropriate affective attitudes; and third, an understanding of the impact of the patient's culture and environment on their condition and their response to it.

## Curricular strategy

Once these educational aims were adopted the unit became involved in a variety of combined teaching projects including the one-month introductory clinical course, the pre-clinical behavioural sciences course, in surgical ward rounds and in paediatric, psychiatric and geriatric clerkships. In 1977 the curriculum committee invited the division 'to explore arranging a regular programme of combined teachings on the third year firms' and this was facilitated by siting the division within the teaching hospital accommodation.

## The clerkship in general practice

The clinical clerkship in general practice began with a fortnight in the student's final year, during which mornings were spent in their tutor's practice, and afternoons in project work and tutorials. Thereafter, a month was included in the penultimate year, in which the second fortnight was spent living in with the doctor. Students received a handbook at the start of the clerkship outlining the educational aims of the attachment and including sections on the distinctive characteristics and content of general practice; communication and data collection and its interpretation; 'extended diagnosis' (clinical, behavioural and ecological); causality and prognosis; and prevention and the theory and practice of screening.

## Other activities

Eight-week student electives were made available for a restricted number of students at the beginning of the final year. In its first year (1974), the division arranged electives for sixteen students, in the UK, North America, West Africa and India. These were intended to provide work experience and to widen the students' views of clinical practice.

One long-term ambition was to combine undergraduate and postgraduate training. Following approval by senate and faculty, a one-year Masters degree course was introduced in 1980 composed of modules on basic statistics, research method, medicine and therapeutics, behavioural science and medical sociology, along with the completion of a research project and dissertation. Six to eight postgraduates attended annually, funded by the DH extended study-leave provision.

Developing research at the same time was a challenge too. The first of the early projects was a three-year study of factors associated with the rejection/early failure of breast feeding, amongst 534 mothers, aimed at enabling the predictive identification of mothers at high risk. The second study was of 222 medical students to test the hypothesis that eight discrete cognitive abilities used in clinical practice can be identified, and their achievement reliably assessed by methods applicable to large numbers of students.

At the end of this first period of the division's life, finance was the major unresolved issue (SIFT money was not yet available). The recruitment of practitioners was severely discouraged by the assigning of their fees and allowances from practice to the university; the salaried income they could achieve was limited, and the tax benefits they had enjoyed as 'self-employed contractors' were no longer available. Inadequate finance also restricted the appointment of research assistants, and this inhibited the development of a systematic divisional research programme in clinical, operational, or demographic aspects of community practice.

Regrettably, developing the relationship between postgraduate training and undergraduate education was never an easy task and its relative failure was the major disappointment of the early years.

## Second generation

With the retirement of John Wright, Leeds medical school decided to give general practice the status of a separate department. At the end of February 1986, Conrad Harris arrived from St Mary's to occupy a new chair, supported by Len Biran (senior lecturer) and Tony Dowell (lecturer) who were already in post. All three had NHS contracts as part-time general practice principals in local practices. The new department was situated in the clinical sciences building at St James' Hospital.

The department now had six weeks in the fourth-year curriculum. There was an introduction to general practice on the first day, then two weeks in a Leeds teaching practice followed by two weeks in a regional teaching practice, and a final fortnight in the department in which the main activities related to consultation skills – using actors and video replay. We were delighted that every year our course was voted by the students as having the best teaching in the fourth year.

Given the small size of the department, research had taken a secondary priority to teaching. Enthusiasm however was fostered by part-time lecturer Alistair Cameron, who with Tony Dowell had interests in early computerised practice management systems. Dowell and Biran also undertook several small-scale research projects in the fields of medical education, mental health and general practice urology. The Masters course that had been started by John Wright continued but was a considerable strain on teaching resources. However, the university was loath to lose the income it brought in. A vocational training scheme was soon set up and proved very popular.

To cope with the growing demands, several part-time appointments were made: Alison Evans, Phil Green and David Adshead, and, from the teaching practices, Arnold Zermansky and Bill Hall. Finally, Jill Thistlethwaite became a full-time senior lecturer in the department for her work on community-based teaching, though the department was not otherwise involved in this. No discussion of our staff would be complete without reference to Lynne Sutton, departmental secretary, and her staff – the backbone of the department.

In 1990, Conrad Harris persuaded the DH that it needed a prescribing research unit (PRU), to take advantage of the national prescribing data collected by the Prescription Pricing Authority in Newcastle. The new unit was set up with a £2m grant and six full-time staff in a Victorian house near the university. Headed by Harris, it produced a large number of reports and many innovative studies during its lifetime. It eventually became a casualty of the DH decision to abandon all its specialist research units, and came to an end in 1996.

In 1993, the department left St James' Hospital and went to another characterful Victorian house in Hyde Terrace near the PRU and the department of epidemiology. It had a much more homely ambiance, and we were very happy with the move. That same year also saw the creation of the Centre for Research in Primary Care (CRPC), with Tony Dowell as the inaugural director. The unit was supported through the academic general practice tasking initiative and received additional support from the Yorkshire RHA. It was located within the research school of medicine, and had a close affiliation with the academic unit of general practice. Its main aim was the promotion and support of primary care research in the old Yorkshire Region. Over the following three years the CRPC developed a number of research streams including clinical trials in areas relevant to primary care (such as H. pylori), HSR, and the development and evaluation of audit in general practice. The CRPC supported early versions of the Yorkshire primary care research group, and the development of a collaborative network of evidence-based primary care teams with the Universities of York, Hull and Newcastle.

The CRPC began building research capacity with the appointment of research fellows Paramjit Gill, now reader in primary care research at Birmingham, and Richard Neal, now professor at the North Wales clinical school. CRPC was also an early promoter of interdisciplinary research, appointing Alison Wilson from a nursing background as the first lecturer in primary care development. Alison Evans took on the running of the Masters course, and Tony Dowell left to take up a chair in New Zealand.

By 1998, when Conrad Harris retired, the department had become, not entirely predictably, a settled, medium-sized constituent of the medical school whose existence was unquestioned – a quiet revolution. Conrad's successor, Phil Heywood, looked to expand the primary care teaching to all stages of the undergraduate curriculum so that medical students could fully realise the extent to which health care was delivered in the community. Len Biran, and his successor Rod Sutcliffe, were keen to involve other health care professionals in the teaching of consultation skills to undergraduate medical students, with Len personally training many of the simulated patients. Other innovations included setting up and running the personal and professional development (PPD) strand which helped raise the profile of general practice and community-based teaching within the medical school, and the establishing of regular support visits to practices taking students. David Pearson joined and helped further expand and integrate the teaching and learning role at both undergraduate and postgraduate level. Robbie Foy was appointed in 2008 as professor of primary care to develop research around implementation medicine.

*John Wright*
*Conrad Harris*
*With thanks to Emma Storr, Jill Thistlethwaite,*
*Bruno Rushforth, Tony Dowell*

# Chapter 12

# The University of Leicester

Leicester was the last of the three new medical schools to be established in the twentieth century after Southampton and Nottingham. It accepted its first medical students in 1975. General practice was initially contained within the department of community health functioning as a semi-autonomous unit alongside epidemiology and biostatistics.

Originally housed on the Leicester Royal Infirmary site, the unit moved to purpose-adapted premises at the Leicester General Hospital in 1992, shortly after becoming an independent department of general practice as a consequence of its widening activities and substantial increase in personnel. In 1995, reflecting its expansion beyond the boundaries of general medical practice, its title was altered to the department of general practice and primary health care. In 2003, following a major reorganisation of the entire medical school into five research departments, the department became the division of general practice and primary health care within the department of health sciences. Staff primarily involved with teaching were transferred to the department of medical and social care education.

The original academic staff consisted of a professor (Marshall Marinker, who left in 1982 to head the MSD Foundation[1]) and five part-time lecturers all on three sessions per week. Four of these went on to more senior positions, namely Robin Fraser (who became a full-time senior lecturer in 1980 and was professor of general practice from 1984–2004), Judith Millac and Henry Patterson (both future regional advisers), and Elan Preston-Whyte (who became a senior lecturer). The practices of these five part-time lecturers became the inner core of a network of more than eighty teaching practices which became the key contributors to our future teaching programmes.

From its inception, academic general practice made a major contribution to undergraduate teaching and assessment. In the early years, general practice was the only discipline which contributed to all five years of the undergraduate curriculum. In years one and two, this consisted of the family placement and agency placement schemes. There was an introductory clinical course of two weeks in year three, and a full-time four-week practice-based course in year four or five, including departmental-based group teaching for one-and-a-half days per week. All students were required to pass the end-of-course examination, which had written and oral components, and was part of the final examination.

Under Marshall Marinker's leadership, Leicester used actors as simulated patients for the teaching of medical students and it became known for its exploration of the doctor–patient relationship. Two outstanding new part-time lecturers were appointed: Brian McAvoy (later professor of general practice successively in Auckland and in Newcastle-upon-Tyne) and Pauline McAvoy (later Dean of education in Auckland before embarking on a distinguished career in NHS management and education).

Under Robin Fraser's leadership, educational activities were strongly focused on the development and assessment of generic consultation skills of undergraduates and on the development and evaluation of teaching and assessment skills of faculty. To aid these activities, department members authored the three editions of *Clinical Method: A General Practice Approach* which became a recommended text in over 75 per cent of UK medical schools and was widely used internationally. Concurrently, a tool for the formative and regulatory assessment of consultation performance, the Leicester Assessment Package (LAP), was developed and evaluated. (Later, similar packages addressing teaching skills and nurse performance were developed and tested.)

In 1990, following widespread curricular reform, the department was given principal responsibility for designing a new integrated course in clinical methods in which all senior clinical students would spend eight weeks full-time in a mix of general practice and hospital settings and with common aims. It was also decided to use the LAP to assess student performance in all clinical examinations (including the final examination which would be hospital-based) and to institute a faculty-wide programme of training courses in teaching and assessment methods for all staff involved in undergraduate teaching and examining. The department was given the task of devising and delivering these training courses and by 2003 over 500 faculty had completed them. Major collaborators in this whole programme were Robin Fraser, Robert McKinley (later professor of general practice at Keele) and Elan Preston-Whyte. Other significant contributors were Adrian Hastings, Gary Aram, Paul Lazarus and Julie Sutton.

Beyond the teaching and educational programmes the department had also extended its range of research interests and by 2003 had expanded to over fifty academic and research staff from medical, nursing, behavioural and social science and IT backgrounds. From a long-term interest and expertise in medical audit methods, the major development was the creation in 1992 of the Eli Lilly National Medical (later Clinical) Audit Centre financed by a 'no-strings' major grant from Eli Lilly. This enabled us to attract Richard Baker to become its director. He developed an extensive programme of research to devise effective methods and guidance to health professionals about improving the quality of care. Due to his expertise in evaluating professional performance, Baker was invited by the CMO to audit the clinical practice of the notorious mass murderer Harold Shipman. Other research themes were HSR led by Andrew Wilson (later a professor) and nursing practice led by Francine Cheater (later professor of nursing research at Leeds).

Following the major school-wide reorganisation in 2002 and Professor Fraser's retirement in 2004, there is no longer a chair in general practice. However, three general practitioners hold chairs within the university (Richard Baker, Kamlesh Khunti and Andrew Wilson), and general practice research remains vibrant, including NIHR programme grants, clinical networks and a Collaboration for Leadership in Applied Health Research and Care (CLAHRC). Adrian Hastings, as a senior clinical educator, is now the general practice educational lead within the department of medical and social care education, and research-active staff have been assigned to the department of health sciences whose head is Richard Baker.

*Robin Fraser*

## Note

1. The MSD Foundation was created in 1982, funded by Merck Sharp and Dohme but academically independent. Between 1983 and 1992 it organised twenty leadership courses for general practitioners.

Chapter 13

# The University of Liverpool

In 1971, the first attempt to create a department of general practice in Liverpool centred on the Palacefields university practice in the then new town of Runcorn, under the directorship of Tony Hall-Turner, previously a general practice principal in Corby. Although modelled on the successful Guy's Hospital development at Thamesmead in London, the Liverpool scheme differed significantly in receiving neither charitable funding nor any financial support from its own medical school, being expected – completely unrealistically – to fund its clinical and academic activities entirely from NHS practice income.

Support from some senior academic staff within the medical school (notably Alastair Breckenridge, the professor of pharmacology and therapeutics), from Pat Byrne (professor of general practice in Manchester), and from Conrad Harris (then a Liverpool general practitioner although about to join the Manchester department as a senior lecturer) was insufficient to match the neutrality – and indeed often active opposition – of other key professors in the medical faculty who were unable to visualise any possibility of a useful role in teaching based in or about general practice.

Despite sterling efforts from the Palacefields principals (Deryck Lambert, Andrew Zurek, Brian McGuinness – then an academic sub-Dean within the faculty of medicine and later professor of general practice at Keele – Jim Newey, Richard Frood and Margaret Upsdell), the venture ended in 1977 when Hall-Turner resigned his position with the university, and the Palacefields practice split into two separate NHS practices, neither formally linked to the medical school.

## A second initiative

The recreation of the department of general practice in 1985 came about following the London Health Planning Consortium's 1981 (Acheson) report on primary health care, which encouraged the view that university departments might influence the standard of local practice and led to significant resource becoming available to universities willing to create this facility. The then Dean of the medical faculty, Sir Robert Shields, saw this as a good opportunity. He was well advised nationally and locally about the necessary critical mass and shape of the proposed department, which was the first of its kind in England not to be substantially dependent on practice NHS income. His concept of clinical leadership alongside non-clinical lectureships was innovative, and has stood the test of time.

There was a groundswell of support in Liverpool from academic and clinical colleagues, including Frank Lowe, the general practice regional adviser, Ian Bogle (then chairman of GMSC), and Alec Stone who headed up the small existing division of general practice within the department of community medicine which had remained as the legacy of the earlier venture and acted primarily as a 'dating agency' between Liverpool students and a few teaching practices, mainly in rural Cheshire. However, support within the faculty of medicine was still equivocal, there being an alternative and influential view from the heads of some of the pre-clinical science departments that the new department should again be based some ten miles off-campus in Runcorn.

Ian Stanley took up his appointment as the foundation professor of general practice in January 1985. His first key decision was to opt decisively for a departmental presence on campus. His second was to offer his clinical services for a week at a time to any practice in Liverpool wishing to use them. In this way he was able, in both faculty and at the RHA, to speak with first-hand knowledge and scotch anecdotal concerns about the standards of local general practice. In addition, he persuaded the Dean that rather than relying on the 'leafy lanes of Cheshire', students could safely be exposed to practice in Liverpool, provided that members of the department could help them to interpret their experience. He also anticipated that the presence of medical students in a wide variety of Liverpool practices would act as a change agent, and help to meet our Acheson remit.

There was sufficient core funding to make three clinical academic appointments – Peter Campion and Peter Bundred as senior lecturers and Susanna Graham-Jones as lecturer – and two non-clinical lectureships in informatics and medical sociology. The latter post was first held by Maggie Pearson and then by Carl May. Despite a potentially serious dispute with local general practitioners over a faculty proposal to house the regional adviser's team within the new department of general practice, and concerns within faculty about appointing clinicians without higher research degrees to senior academic posts, the new department was generally well received by both town and gown. Ian Stanley was made faculty representative on Liverpool RHA.

The faculty was generous with curriculum time for the new department, especially when one considers quite how traditional the undergraduate curriculum was in the 1980s. Both the new non-clinical lecturers contributed to introductory courses in year one and had their own behavioural science lecture courses. We pioneered project work on teams and about 'mental health in the community', both innovative (if sometimes overwhelming!) undertakings. Our third-year clinical course, while still largely experiential, introduced new methods of personal objective setting, communication skills training and of assessment. As a direct result, when Liverpool decided on wholesale medical curriculum reform in the early 1990s, we were part of the small group in faculty leading this process.

The department began to expand in the late 1980s with the benefit of part-time outside-funded (ICI Stuart) research fellowships for clinical colleagues, and two externally funded lectureships in management (Wellcome) and in medical ethics (Health Education Authority). The latter was subsequently consolidated into a university-funded post, in part to support our new Masters in medical ethics. Research income started to flow, and the department successfully hosted the annual AUTGP meeting in 1989. Chris Dowrick joined the department in 1991. As a result of expansion in national and regional funding streams for academic general practice, two additional junior clinical academic posts were created in the early 1990s (held by Frances Mair and Karen Fairhurst), confirming that the department of general practice in Liverpool was now an established entity.

*Brian McGuinness*
*Ian Stanley*
*Christopher Dowrick*

# Chapter 14

# The University of Manchester

## The intellectual environment

During the 1930s, John Ryle's philosophy of 'social medicine' was developed. Its central tenet was that illness should be studied in relation to the patient's occupational and social environment. These beliefs were held by Fraser Brockington, who became the Manchester professor of social and preventive medicine, and by Robert Platt, the professor of medicine. A social medicine 'laboratory' was required and the then Vice-Chancellor, John Stopford, set about finding one. A suitable building for an experimental health centre was found close to the university.

## Darbishire House

Stopford secured grants from the Rockefeller and Nuffield foundations to buy Darbishire House for £17,500 in 1950. All that was needed was some general practitioners to bring their practices into it. The local general practitioners worked single-handed and, with a declining population, were in fierce competition with each other for patients. However, after many meetings, Drs Ashworth, Goldie, Lenten and Davies agreed to move in, reassured by the financial arrangements offered and places on the management committee. Darbishire House Health Centre, with its own laboratory and X-ray facilities, opened in 1954. To facilitate research Bob Logan was appointed reader to liaise between the practice and the department of social and preventive medicine.

## The establishment of the department

By the early 1960s Manchester students were being attached to general practitioners throughout the region, mostly to practices recommended by the north-west RCGP faculty. Pat Byrne's practice in Milnthorpe was one of them. He complained to John Stopford that the school never asked him about the students he taught, or them about the teaching they got. It was arranged that he should see Robert Platt, and the upshot was that he joined the steering committee considering teaching in general practice. In 1965 he was appointed part-time lecturer in the department of medicine, continuing to practice in Milnthorpe. In 1968 he was appointed full-time senior lecturer. That year Drs Lenten, Goldie and Davies all retired, allowing the appointment of Bill Acheson and John Wright as senior lecturers and Rodney Wilkin as lecturer. Henry Ashworth remained an honorary lecturer. In 1969 general practice became an independent department with Byrne as its director, and in 1971 he was promoted to professor of general practice, the first in England. In 1970, Eileen Ineson, a psychiatric social worker, was appointed as a lecturer with a clinical role in the practice.

## The Byrne years

At this time undergraduate teaching consisted of a two-week attachment in the third (first clinical) year to one of the twelve 'inner ring' practices which Pat Byrne had recruited. There was a seminar at each end (the first being mainly to inform students about the practices they would be going to, the second to discuss their experiences). For some students this would be their first clinical experience. In their fourth year students were attached to district general hospitals throughout the region and while there had a two-week attachment to local practices. The department had little control over what they were taught or how.

Byrne, a leading light in the RCGP education committee which was refining educational objectives and methods, made contact with the faculty of education, through which he met Barrie Long. With Long he ran a series of courses for teachers, initially directed at general practice undergraduate teachers, but later directed at general practice trainers. Together they developed small-group teaching and published *Learning to Care, Person to Person*. Byrne recruited Jim Freeman, an educational psychologist, as a research associate to study vocational training which was just getting under way. For these studies the Manchester department was awarded the status of a chief scientist's research unit.

Byrne and Long also recorded and analysed verbal behaviours in the consultations, resulting in their book *Doctors Talking to Patients*. Acheson also had DHSS funding for a study on the doctor-patient relationship and later for a survey of general practitioners' educational needs (which highlighted the shortcomings of their undergraduate education in particular with reference to teaching methods). He was also funded by the RHA for a study on the cost of illness. Gareth Lloyd used data from his Oldham practice for some descriptive research, while Wilkin got an MD (then rare for general practitioners) for his studies on alcoholism using the Darbishire House practice as his laboratory. Conrad Harris developed teaching in consultation skills using actors and video playback and completed his Masters in education before going to London and later to the chair in Leeds. He was replaced by Bernard Marks, a general practitioner from Salford with an interest in asthma. Alex Brown joined the department from his practice in the north-east.

## The next phase

Pat Byrne retired in 1978 and was succeeded by David Metcalfe who had been senior lecturer (general practice) in community health at Nottingham. A little later, Gareth Lloyd left and was replaced by Idris Williams, who had gained an MD for his studies of care for elderly people in his Bolton practice, and Carl Whitehouse joined the department from his practice in Lewes.

In 1982 the department and practice moved from Darbishire House into Rusholme Health Centre, a purpose-built premises in Walmer Street, which meant a considerable change in the patient population. The newly named 'Robert Darbishire Practice' took advantage of the DHSS 'Micros for general practitioners' scheme to explore what computers could do, and under Carl Whitehouse's leadership with Margaret Flynn (the practice manager), the ABIES system was installed. In 1986 Ashworth and Acheson retired and Whitehouse won promotion to senior lecturer when Williams was appointed to the chair at Nottingham.

Although it had been made clear that the curriculum was fixed, David Metcalfe was able to introduce communication-skills teaching using professional actors from 'Northwest Spanner' led by Penny Morris, joint ward rounds with some consultants, and community follow up where students visited a patient they had clerked at their homes after discharge, reporting back to a seminar led by the consultant concerned and a general practitioner tutor. However these experiences were patchy over the three teaching hospitals.

In 1986, after four years of negotiation, an eight-week multidisciplinary module based on the human life cycle was introduced. The other departments involved were public health, occupational health and geriatric medicine, with some paediatric time. The overlap between subjects as evidenced by the patients they saw increased effective teaching time. However the multidisciplinary seminars required teaching skills and professionalism that were not always provided by the other departments. While the professor of child health, Robert Boyd, approved of learning about children in their homes and families, Raymond Tallis, who succeeded John Brocklehurst as professor of geriatric medicine, insisted that the care of the aged was taught in hospital, so the module disintegrated. Because all the module teaching took place in Manchester inner ring practices, the general practitioners in the region who had provided the fourth-year attachments were stood down, which they did not like!

When Metcalfe succeeded Byrne the department's status as a chief scientist's research unit was continued, but he was told he need not confine himself to the educational subjects that Byrne and Freeman had pursued. He had already determined to investigate any contribution that general practitioners might make to the inequality in morbidity and mortality that John Brotherston had reported in his 1975 Galton Lecture. Following Donabedian, he determined to survey 'structure' (premises, equipment, staff and the like), 'process' (actions taken in the consultation) and 'outcome' (in this case the subjective health status of people in the study area). To do this he recruited Jo Wood and David Wilkin as senior research fellows, David later becoming associate director. Ralph Leavey was recruited as research fellow and Lesley Hallam as research co-ordinator (later unit manager).

Seventy-six per cent of principals in Greater Manchester (396 out of 522) agreed to be interviewed in their practices for the 'structure' study. This showed that the inner city was well served; the poorest practices were in the inner suburbs nearby. Of these doctors, 208 took part in the 'process' study, collecting data on one of each weekdays in each quarter of the year. This produced 140,000 consultations to analyse, and they showed a social-class gradient, upper-class patients being more likely to be referred or investigated and less likely to get a prescription. Importantly there were wide variations between doctors for these rates. The variations between individual doctors, much greater within areas than between areas, raised questions about their effects on patients and the outcomes of care.

At the same time, interviews with 1,900 people about their health showed that while people in the lower social classes had poorer subjective health as measured with the Nottingham Health Profile they only consulted at the same rate as those in higher classes.

Several members of the clinical staff used this data for their own studies, Clare Ronalds on the work of women doctors, Paul Hodgkin on diagnostic clusters, Whitehouse on the management of psychosocial illness and Williams on the care of the elderly. Hallam got an MSc for her studies of telephone use by general practitioners. Colin Bradley, later professor at Cork, got an MD for his study of uncertainty in prescribing.

## Major change

Three successive Deans (Leslie Turnberg, Robert Boyd and Steve Tomlinson) were concerned to implement major change in the under-graduate curriculum. David Metcalfe had been heavily involved in some early working parties and in 1991 was invited to give his services fully to curriculum development. A proleptic appointment to the chair was proposed. Martin Roland was appointed, taking up the position full-time from August 1992. Metcalfe left his full-time post the follow-ing January, although he remained part-time as adviser on curriculum development until retiring three years later. Carl Whitehouse continued the major involvement in the educational field as the new problem-based learning curriculum, based on broad systems rather than departmental disciplines, came into being from 1994 with much greater general prac-tice and community involvement (one-fifth of curricular time in years three to five). He was promoted professor of teaching medicine in the community, the first such appointment in the UK.

Acknowledging that 'outcomes' research was in its infancy in this country, the research unit (now the Centre for Primary Care Research, or CPCR) started a new programme with a critical review of instru-ments available to measure outcomes in primary care. It went on to look at quality measures, and in due course joined with other university departments and groups from the Universities of York and Salford to bid for the government funded National Primary Care Research and Development Centre (NPCRDC). This bid was successful and NPCRDC came into being in 1995. David Wilkin became chief executive and Martin Roland became director of research and development.

NPCRDC became a separate department and moved out of Rusholme Health Centre, separating clinical from research staff. By 1998 the concept of small departments was being seen as inappropriate, particu-larly in the research field, so the medical school became a single depart-ment. Within this a school of primary care emerged, headed by Roland

and including NPCRDC, the Robert Darbishire Practice, and what was known as the 'Rusholme Academic Unit' with its own small area of clinical and educational research and responsibility for teaching.

Following the merging of the Victoria University of Manchester with UMIST in 2004, the new Manchester University had four faculties. Within the faculty of medical and human sciences, the school of medicine was divided into the Manchester medical school responsible for clinical education, with Val Wass (who had succeeded Whitehouse) as professor of community-based medical education, and four research schools. The primary care research group was located within the health sciences research group in the school of community-based medicine, and NPCRDC (whose contract with government ended at the end of 2010 after fifteen fulfilling years) was seen as academically independent. Martin Roland left NPCRDC in 2009 to return to Cambridge. As from June 2010 the university relinquished control of the Robert Darbishire Practice and the experiment of the 1950s was completed.

*David Metcalfe*
*Carl Whitehouse*

# Chapter 15

# The University of Newcastle

The medical school in Newcastle had its origins in a series of lectures organised by a group of local practitioners beginning in 1832. Of the eight students enrolled, John Snow was to become the most distinguished, removing the handle of the Broad Street pump and becoming anaesthetist to Queen Victoria at the birth of two of her children in the 1850s. By 1834 the popularity of the lectures led to the foundation of the Newcastle College of Medicine which by 1851 had established a close connection with the developing University of Durham, allowing the College to award Durham degrees in 1856. In 1934 Durham College united with Armstrong College to become King's College in the University of Durham, continuing until 1963 until separation again occurred when the University of Newcastle upon Tyne (now the University of Newcastle) was established.

Medical teaching was in the hands of clinicians with honorary university appointments. When Newcastle's first medical officer of health was appointed in 1870, public health teaching began on a similar honorary basis. While the development of the laboratory disciplines led slowly to the creation of full-time posts, similar clinical appointments were rarely achieved until after the Second World War – and there were none in public health.

## 1964: Family and community medicine

This was the situation in 1960 when the first of several curriculum reviews began. Andrew Smith, a Foundation Council member of the College of General Practitioners, together with Roland Freedman and H.G. 'Bingy' Barnes, had begun sensitising members of the faculty of medicine to the potential of general practice education. The new curriculum, due to begin in 1962, provided the opportunity. Based on the principles of integration and early clinical experience, planning became the responsibility of a multiplicity of committees, one of which was entitled family and social medicine. Chaired by Donald Court, James Spence's successor to the chair of child health, including Richard Pearson (the medical officer of health and honorary lecturer in public health), R. C. Browne (the professor of industrial health) and others, and consulting with local general practitioners including Keith Hodgkin and Aubrey Colling, the committee devised a four-week experimental course in family and community medicine in which placements in general practice alternated each week with experience in community services. It was recommended that the course required the urgent appointment of a senior lecturer in public health with the future appointment of a lecturer in general practice.

John Walker, previously lecturer in general practice in the Edinburgh department, was appointed lecturer in public health in July 1964 with the aim of starting the course in October. No other steps to implement the plan had been taken. Within three months, twelve local general practitioners were appointed tutors in family medicine (within the department of medicine in deference to attitudes to public health). Community staff were selected and briefed and six hospital consultants, invited at the suggestion of the general practitioners, were to act as mentors. This inspired suggestion created a unique teaching group, ultimately demonstrating the huge potential of general practice to every clinical discipline in the faculty of medicine. Popular with both students and staff, the four weeks were extended to five once the experimental period ended, the course becoming an integral part of the curriculum[1] and attracting international interest and many visitors from the UK and overseas. Meanwhile the department of public health continued to teach social and preventive medicine and, until 1968 when NHS changes cast doubts on its future, a course leading to the diploma in public health.

In 1969 Richard Pearson retired and John Walker, who had been promoted to senior lecturer, was appointed head of a re-titled department of family and community medicine. During these years the number of general practitioner tutors had increased, consultants had rotated, the teaching group had developed clear aims and become cohesive, and tutors were now pleased to have their university posts within the new department of family and community medicine.

The establishment of the new department coincided with the creation of the medical care research unit in collaboration with the department of medical statistics (later to become the Centre for Health Services Research) in which early work included the study of patients' attitudes to A&E departments, general practice/hospital relationships, and the early care of infants with spina bifida, the results of which influenced national policy.

These developments coincided with the department's role in establishing and developing vocational training in collaboration with the regional postgraduate institute. In 1969, the initial three-year programme based on seven teaching practices began, after negotiation to allow division of the trainee year into two six-month periods. Andrew Smith was appointed part-time lecturer in the department to provide direction and co-ordination. The programme[2] continued within the department until becoming part of the regional adviser network.

When the RCGP established its examination in 1968, Andrew Smith and John Walker were among the early examiners. When Walker became examination secretary in 1972, members of the department and the university computing laboratory played an increasing role in its development.

A second curriculum review in 1974 led to further innovation in the form of the groundbreaking multidisciplinary course in human development, behaviour and ageing. Notable features were the integrated approach, visits to a general practice surgery, and the community-based family study in the first year and patient study in the second year, in which members of the department provided orientation and continuity through leadership of permanent tutorial groups.[3]

John Walker was awarded a personal chair in 1976 and in 1977 when the revised curriculum was introduced, the university made additional appointments of several part-time lecturers and two full-time senior lecturers – Don Foster to become responsible for postgraduate teaching and research in community medicine and Chris Drinkwater in family medicine with the aim of developing a university teaching practice. He joined Krish Kumar, an elderly single-handed practitioner based in Benwell, one of Newcastle's deprived areas. The practice moved from its run-down premises to a local shopping centre in 1984 when it was opened by Donald Acheson who was then CMO. In turn when the shopping centre was to be demolished, Chris masterminded the funding and development of the purpose-built West End Resource Centre which included the Adelaide Medical Centre opened in 1996 by Tony Blair, then leader of the Opposition. Throughout this time the practice was funded almost entirely from NHS sources. The practitioners held academic appointments and four have since been appointed to chairs.

Increased staffing of the department was achieved in 1985 by the appointment of two senior lectureships in community medicine. Research, particularly in prescribing, continued. The department established a local and national profile in service development areas as diverse as care of the elderly, clinical audit and teamwork. International projects included training general practitioners and nurse trainers in the Basque region of Spain, and training and examining general practitioners in Kuwait.

In 1988 John Walker retired and the department became two divisions, primary care and epidemiology and public health, marking the start of a series of titular and organisational changes in the faculty and university.

## Primary health care

The William Leech chair of primary care was established in 1990, with Roger Jones its first incumbent in 1991. The first chair in epidemiology and public health was also established, and Raj Bhopal appointed. Both made significant contributions to developing research. When Roger Jones moved to the chair at UMDS in 1993, Chris Drinkwater became acting head until the appointment of Brian McAvoy in 1994. Brian stayed for five years before returning to Australia.

In the 1994 curriculum review, primary health care was again central. Indeed the faculty turned to the department for guidance and leadership in developing topics such as communication skills and ethics, which had been pioneered in the human development, behaviour and ageing course from 1977 onwards. Now over 130 practices in the region were involved in teaching. A service-based clinical rotation in public health was also introduced, one of the first of its kind in the UK. The most recent curriculum review in 2001, paralleling a significant increase in student numbers and a new partnership with the University of Durham, saw further expansion of community-based teaching and a personal chair in primary care and medical education for John Spencer. Some 230 practices are currently involved with general practice input to all years of the curriculum, and the teaching region stretches from the Scottish borders across to the Lakes and down to the north Yorks moors, including the three great river conurbations of Tyneside, Wearside and Teesside. Feedback from students about general practice teaching remains consistently positive.

In 2002 major restructuring took place within the university with the dissolution of departments, the reorganisation of schools and the creation of (research) institutes. Paradoxically, the university, having been one of the first English medical schools to establish a department of general practice, became the first to dissolve one. General practice and public health teaching in the early years of the curriculum and primary care research stayed within the school of population and health sciences which later became the Institute of Health and Society. Martin Eccles was appointed William Leech professor of primary care research. Clinical teaching in general practice relocated to the school of medical sciences education development. The Adelaide Medical Centre separated from the university administration and reverted to being run by the PCT as an ordinary general practice, although remaining involved in teaching.

To date all aspects of academic enterprise that started out under the heading of family and community medicine remain alive and well, albeit operating in different contexts and locations within the faculty but lacking the visibility and identity they enjoyed when under one roof. Nevertheless, community-based subjects have achieved high ratings in recent RAEs. The research portfolio spans clinical effectiveness, aspects of ageing including the impact of dementia, clinical decision-making, environmental epidemiology, as well as major involvement in the Newcastle Clinical Trials Unit. Primary health care and public health have also consistently made significant contributions to the success of recent teaching quality audits.

On these grounds it would seem that the uncontrolled experiment initiated over forty-five years ago has been a resounding success.

*John Walker*
*John Spencer*

## Notes

1. Walker J.H. and Barnes H.G., 'Teaching of family and community medicine', *BMJ*, 2, 1966: 1129–30.
2. Special correspondent, 'Vocational training in general practice. II. Newcastle upon Tyne', *BMJ*, 2, 1971: 763–5.
3. Forster D.P., Drinkwater C.K., Corradine A., and Cowley K., 'The family study: a model for integrating the individual and community perspective in medical education', *Medical Education*, 26, 1992: 110–15.

# Chapter 16

# The University of Nottingham

## The beginnings

The University of Nottingham received its Charter in 1948, but it was some time before it had a medical school. By the late 1960s agreement was reached between the then Sheffield Regional Hospital Board and the university that there should be a university teaching hospital in Nottingham which allowed the university to proceed with the founding of a medical school. The first forty-eight students were admitted in September 1970 and the faculty was officially inaugurated in October 1970 by Sir Keith Joseph, the Secretary of State for Health and Social Services. Responsibility for general practice teaching was placed in the department of community health led by its Professor Maurice Backett.

## The development

There was no general practice teaching until the first students entered the clinical part of their courses in May 1973. By this time five part-time general practice lecturers had been recruited each with an honorarium to acknowledge their contribution. They included Alan Murphy, John Skinner, Tom Venables, Peter Sprackling and Harold Lee. David Metcalfe was appointed senior lecturer in 1972. He had experience of British general practice in Yorkshire and had been teaching and practising family medicine in Rochester, USA.

In 1975 Noeline McCoach and Jim McCracken were appointed part-time lecturers and Mike Sheldon also joined the team as senior lecturer. The teaching group was given full autonomy in the development of undergraduate teaching in general practice. They met regularly every Wednesday afternoon in huts on the university campus described with some derision as 'cowsheds'. The standard of medicine practised by the group was high and the lecturers were much respected by the students. David Metcalfe quoted Edmund Burke as saying 'Example is the school of mankind, and they will learn at no other.' Certainly the learning opportunity allowed by being in the surgery with the general practitioner was good.

## An independent department at last

By the end of the 1970s the university hospital and medical school buildings were completed. They were part of a single complex known as The Queen's Medical Centre. The department of community medicine moved to its new home in the medical school. Professor Backett had moved on and been replaced by Professor Mark Ellwood. By this time David Metcalfe had also departed to take up the chair of general practice in Manchester following the retirement of Professor Byrne. This was a blow to his colleagues. In their opinion it put full autonomy for general practice in Nottingham back considerably. In particular Alan Murphy deserves recognition for the work he did in making a compelling case for an independent department professorially led. In 1985 the university decided that there should be an independent department of general practice. I was privileged to take up the appointment of foundation chair in general practice on 1 October 1985. The chair and two senior lecturers were funded with UGC money.

## Early years

I inherited a skilled and dedicated group of lecturers and administrative staff. The teaching was of a high order. The linkage between the 'in practice' learning and that provided in small groups in the school was excellently co-ordinated. Each student had a handbook which set out clear objectives as well as information about seminars, projects, audits and simulated patient teaching.

Mike Pringle was promoted senior lecturer as was Tom O'Dowd from Cardiff. Other appointments followed and the newly formed department quickly became functional. There was an increase in research activity and postgraduate teaching. Medical audit spread throughout the county (I was chair of the Medical Audit Advisory Board) and good relations were built with Nottingham FHSA.

## Curriculum development

In 1991 the faculty board commissioned a curricular review working party. From the start, years one and two of the course had comprised three themes. One was basically physiology; another anatomy; and the third covered the community. A fourth theme was introduced termed 'personal and professional development'. This had originated in the department of general practice and was now fully absorbed into the curriculum.

Being introduced to patients and their problems at an early stage in training certainly encouraged personal and professional development. General practice was well placed to develop this and take responsibility for its management.

## Further developments

Interesting events have happened since my retirement. Tony Avery has been head of division since 1998 and now shares the role with Denise Kendrick. The school of community health sciences now includes divisions of epidemiology and public health, primary care, rehabilitation and ageing, and psychiatry, and was headed for six years by Mike Pringle.

The division of primary care has an increasing role in undergraduate and postgraduate education, and a growing portfolio of high quality research. There are now five professors in the division and senior academics have developed strong research teams with support from major funding bodies, particularly the NIHR. The development of the department was built on research. My research in care of the elderly was supplemented by Tom O'Dowd's on 'heartsink' patients. Mike Pringle researched quality assurance (notably significant event audits) and with Julia Hippisley-Cox set up an epidemiological research database. Tony Avery has contributed to improved patient safety in the field of prescribing, and Denise Kendrick is an expert in accident prevention. In the last RAE, primary care research was the highest rated in the medical school. The division is now a member of the NIHR English national school for primary care research.

Academic general practice has come a long way since 1970, and the setting up of a separate department in 1985, and there is every sign that the discipline will continue to flourish.

*Idris Williams*

# Chapter 17

# The University of Oxford

The origins of the University of Oxford are said to be 'lost in the mists of antiquity'. It is thought to date from the mid-twelfth century with the migration of students from Paris. 'Physic' was one of the early subjects studied, with a status approaching that of theology!

Formal teaching of medical sciences to undergraduates did not start until the end of the nineteenth century, when chairs of anatomy and physiology were established. Clinical teaching was regarded by the university as a 'trade' and was left to the London teaching hospitals. An eventual change in this attitude was fortuitous, though there was much resistance both from medical science tutors in Oxford Colleges and from consultants in local hospitals. In the late 1930s Lord Nuffield (of motor car fame) offered substantial funds to establish a handful of clinical medical professorships. After prolonged negotiation, these funds were accepted by the university, albeit with reluctance. This was the beginning of the Oxford clinical school. It facilitated another circumstantial event – the evacuation of some clinical students from London teaching hospitals to Oxford to escape the bombing of London in the early 1940s.

I came to Oxford in 1950 as an undergraduate to do four years 'medical sciences' (we were discouraged from calling ourselves medical students). When the decision about 'clinical' was made it was assumed I would go to a London teaching hospital, recommended by my College tutor. I went to University College Hospital and only six of my year of about seventy students stayed on in Oxford – and these for domestic reasons such as being married and having families.

I returned to Oxford as a general practitioner in 1959 and found things were changing, with plans for a big new hospital (the John Radcliffe) strengthening arguments for the establishment of a major clinical school. More and more students stayed in Oxford to do their clinical and by 1970 nearly all were doing this. But it took almost a decade more for general practice to get into the clinical course.

Sir Richard Doll's appointment as Regius professor of medicine in 1970 changed things. He was determined to get both public health and general practice into the curriculum. A chair of public health was established in 1974 but there was much more debate about general practice. Finally, resistance was overcome, though the commitment was minimal, and in 1977 a part-time readership in general practice was established within the department of social and community medicine.

This post was to be combined with being a half-time principal in a local general practice. Funding for five years came from the RHA. Although I was strongly supportive of the initiative and had assisted in its achievement, I was disappointed with the 'token' outcome. As a full-time local general practitioner of twenty years standing with limited teaching experience and minimal research training I felt unqualified for the job myself. But I was persuaded to apply and was told I had an overriding asset – the respect and support of local general practitioners. I was offered the job and accepted with considerable foreboding, especially as there was no support except a part-time secretary.

The first few years were a painful experience. Changing from being a full-time to a part-time general practitioner was difficult for patients, for practice colleagues and for me. Establishing student teaching was hard work and I was grateful to general practice academic colleagues in other universities for guidance and help. But the most important help came from general practice colleagues in and around Oxford who were willing to have students in their practices. Without too much difficulty, I recruited about seventy practices from the Oxford region to take a student for a residential two-week attachment at the beginning of the clinical course. A bigger challenge was the selection of eight practices in or very close to Oxford with a university-appointed tutor in each. These practices were required to take eight final-year students a year, each for two weeks. Tutors were also required to participate in teaching and meetings in the department. Remuneration was paltry – £250 annually for each practice from a trust fund!

After two years, we all agreed that tutors deserved more funding. A bid was developed and submitted to the medical school. When this was rejected, the tutors and I tendered our resignations. This action, along with a survey which showed how much medical students valued general practice teaching, resulted in tutors being offered a proper sessional fee and the university took over payment for the part-time readership. Our resignations were withdrawn. Soon after this, we were awarded a Jephcott visiting professorship by the RCGP and John Fry accepted the appointment with enthusiasm. His weekly visit was a great boost to the morale of general practitioner teachers and his valedictory lecture took to task the medical faculty for their failure to properly support our embryonic general practice department.

Meanwhile, a research programme evolved slowly. It focused on prevention, health promotion and smoking cessation, with funding from the Health Education Council, the British Heart Foundation and other medical charities. Funding for two part-time lectureships came from outside moneys, and the establishment in the department by the ICRF (now Cancer Research UK) of its General Practice Research Group was greatly welcomed.

By the early 1990s the general practice side of what had become the department of public health and primary care was thriving and it was time to bid for a chair and a properly structured and funded department, especially in the light of the increasing teaching demands made by the medical school to implement prevailing GMC recommendations. This bid was accepted. It was agreed that, with my approaching retirement, there should be a fully funded statutory professor of general practice (to supplement the readership). It was also agreed that the department would become a department of primary care, independent from the department of public health. In the meantime, I was appointed ad hominem professor.

I retired in 1997 and for one year general practice was headed by Martin Lawrence, for many years a part-time university lecturer in general practice (along with Theo Schofield) but now terminally ill. In 1998, David Mant was appointed professor of general practice and head of an independent department of primary health care, with Tim Lancaster as reader. This increase in senior critical mass was a key breakthrough, allowing the professor to develop the research programme while Tim Lancaster, who also became the medical school's director of clinical studies (clinical Dean), developed the teaching programme.

Becoming a separate department allowed the establishment of research in vascular disease, childhood infection and patient experience and the development of a research agenda to provide evidence to underpin clinical general practice. It also facilitated a more extensive student teaching programme. Since the fragile beginning in 1977 it had taken more than twenty years to achieve this solid base!

In 2005–2006 the growing importance of general-practice-led research was recognised when the government-funded national school for health research decided to establish a national school for primary care research, which the five departments of primary care (including Oxford) in England which had performed best in the 2001 RAE were invited to form. The success of this initiative has since led to an expansion in the educational role and the school is now tasked with ensuring that the

UK maintains its international leadership in primary care research by training the next generation of world-class researchers.

*Godfrey Fowler*

I am grateful to my successor, David Mant, for bringing this account up-to-date. He, in turn, retired in 2009 but the university has, true to form, still not made a replacement appointment a year later, so he remains acting head!

# Chapter 18

# The University of Sheffield

## First steps

As in other medical schools, general practice emerged in Sheffield as a distinct academic discipline from under the umbrella of community medicine. In the 1950s and 1960s, final-year medical students had a two-day attachment for six weeks in general practice as part of the public health placement, organised by the then department of social medicine.

In 1972, Eric Wilkes was appointed to the new chair of general practice within the department of community medicine headed by John Knowelden. There were several local applicants for the chair, but Eric Wilkes was a well-known local general practitioner in Baslow, who had recently founded St Luke's Hospice, the first of its kind outside London. Three associates in general practice were also appointed on a sessional basis, namely Simon Barley, Helen Joesbury and David Dalrymple-Smith.

Professor Wilkes remained medical director of St Luke's for fifteen years, combining this with his academic post. Initially he continued as a partner in the Baslow practice, but his other responsibilities made this impossible to maintain. He was responsible for questions on general practice in the degree examination for community medicine, and for organising student attachments, including to St Luke's, and to a family with a new baby. This latter was at first voluntary, but later became part of the curriculum as the family attachment scheme. He also started a series of postgraduate lectures for general practitioners.

Professor Wilkes, a popular lecturer, considerably raised the profile of general practice in the medical school. Partly due to the university's need to save money, he retired in 1983, and the post remained vacant for four years. During the interregnum, student attachments were organised by general practitioners, at first Malcolm Taylor and then Alan Evans, who had sessional appointments in the department of community medicine under Professor Brian Williams.

During his time, Wilkes tried to establish a university practice, for which funds were set aside, at the Northern General Hospital. But this failed to materialise, as did another attempt to attract a new professor as a partner to a practice in Crookes. At the time there were two models for university departments of general practice. One was practice-based where academic staff were partners in a university teaching practice, and the other was practice-linked where university staff had clinical appointments in different practices. Initially, the practice-based departments were the largest and most successful. But this model became increasingly difficult for academic clinical staff to maintain, with more stringent requirements for partnerships from the NHS on the one hand, and more recently pressure from the university RAEs.

## The second chair appointment

In 1987, a new professor, David Hannay, was appointed as a full-time university employee, and was left to make his own clinical arrangements. He joined a practice at the Park Health Centre as a partner, at first full-time and then part-time doing three clinical sessions a week. Hannay came from a rural practice in south-west Scotland, having previously been a senior lecturer in the department in Glasgow. His interests were in illness behaviour, medical sociology and medical education, having been a research fellow at McMaster University.

As the only full-time member of a sub-department within the department of community medicine, Hannay's priorities were to achieve a critical mass of academic staff and to develop undergraduate teaching in the new curriculum. Four general practitioners with three sessions a week (Paul Hodgkin, Helen Joesbury, John Poyser and Nigel Shanks) were appointed from UGC funding to undertake teaching and develop their own research. In addition, a lecturer in medical sociology (Nick Fox) was partly funded from Professor Hannay's practice earnings.

The sub-department was still considerably understaffed in relation to other medical schools of similar size, and in recognition of this a senior lecturer (Tim Usherwood) was appointed along with a part-time secretary to support Diane Allen, the departmental secretary. The sub-department was also successful in obtaining two research fellowships from the RCGP, and a senior research fellow funded jointly with the department of psychiatry. The director of St Lukes (Dr Crowther) and the postgraduate adviser (Dr Rees-Jones) were appointed as honorary lecturers.

As a result of this expansion, the sub-department became a full department in 1989, within an academic division of community medicine which included the renamed department of public health medicine and the medical care research unit. In order to accommodate the growing department, funds originally set aside for a university practice were used to build an extension on to a flat roof space in the medical school at the Royal Hallamshire Hospital. This was opened in 1992, and additional part-time lecturers were appointed (Amanda Howe, Caroline Mitchell and Paul Wilson). In 1994, the department moved to refurbished premises on two floors of the community sciences centre at the Northern General Hospital, and subsequently to the adjacent Samuel Fox House.

The department was now teaching throughout the revised curriculum, with first aid and a family attachment scheme linked to medical sociology in the first year, a short course on communication skills in the third year, and a five-week module in the final year incorporating self-directed learning and continuous assessment which counted towards the degree examination. The teaching relied on about ninety honorary clinical tutors in the community and the administrative skills of departmental secretaries. It was favourably reviewed by the GMC and now comprises almost one fifth of the undergraduate curriculum.

In 1991 a successful multidisciplinary Masters course in primary and community care was established, and in 1992 an additional senior lecturer (Nigel Mathers) and non-clinical lecturer (Peggy Newton) were funded by the Trent RHA. By 1993, four members of the department had obtained doctorates by research, with two others matriculated for an MD and two more for an MPhil. In addition, the department had attracted five research fellowships and four postgraduate research students. Departmental staff were also teaching courses on research methods in both the medical and nursing schools. By 1995, the department of general practice included the secretary of the Sheffield faculty of the RCGP, and the administrator for the Sheffield medical audit advisory group. In addition, the postgraduate adviser in general practice (Donald Fairclough) was part of the department, thus beginning to integrate undergraduate and postgraduate general practice.

In 1996, the pressures of the RAE led to the establishment of the school of health and related research (ScHARR) to which the department of general practice was moved from the medical school. This was resisted by Professor Hannay, who argued that it was not appropriate to remove a department representing half of all doctors from a medical school. Hannay left the chair of general practice after ten years to return to rural practice in Scotland and run a regional primary care research network. During his time, academic general practice in Sheffield had become established and three senior lecturers had become professors, namely Tim Usherwood in Sydney, Amanda Howe in East Anglia, and Nigel Mathers who succeeded Hannay in Sheffield.

### Further developments

In 1997, the department of general practice became the Institute of General Practice and Primary Care (IGPPC). Professor Mathers was the director, with a remit to develop a primary care research culture within ScHARR, along with Dr Moyez Jiwa as research co-ordinator and Dr Gary Butler as teaching co-ordinator. A knowledge transfer pro-gramme was developed under Robert Glendenning. IGPPC expanded to more than 100 members of staff. Professor Mathers led four European projects culminating in the establishment of a network of European general practitioners in Poland, Belgium, Italy, Spain, Slovenia, Czech Republic and Switzerland which provided the basis for the *European Textbook of Family Medicine* (2006).

Most of the IGPPC staff were non-clinical and much of its research had little appeal for general practitioners. The non-clinical researchers expected academic general practice to provide patients for clinical trials but this was not what general practitioners had joined the IGPPC to do. Thus in 2006 the Institute returned to the medical school as the Academic Unit of Primary Medical Care (AUPMC), leaving behind the majority of the non-clinical members of the IGPPC who felt their academic careers were best served by remaining within the non-clinical school. However, prior to the transfer of the IGPPC clinicians to the medical school, a strong argument was made that the research and teaching components of general practice should be divided, with the researchers remaining in the non-clinical school and the teaching functions being transferred to medical education. This was resisted since for the discipline to continue to develop it was important to recognise that teaching and research are mutually dependent.

The other issue which was addressed was the historical discontinu-ity between the undergraduate and postgraduate elements of general practice training with the result that the former is funded by HEFC and the latter by the NHS. Although the local NHS deanery supported the move of AUPMC out of the non-clinical school and the transfer of clini-cians into the medical school, the local board of the RCGP decided to remain within the non-clinical school despite the fact that Paul Wilson, convenor of the RCGP oral examination, and Professor Mathers, chair of the national RCGP clinical innovation and research centre were senior members of the AUPMC.

Shortly after, an external review recommended that AUPMC should become a larger primary care unit containing a better balance of clinical and non-clinical staff and an improved research environment. A new research and teaching strategy was developed in response to this review with a focus on translational research ('translating evidence into practice') and translational teaching ('putting teaching theory into practice'). Subsequently, AUPMC moved into modern accommodation in Samuel Fox House to be co-located with the school of nursing. Henry Smithson was appointed acting head of unit in 2010 and established the 'CUTLER' group of fourteen research practices in South Yorkshire as part of the NIHR primary care research network. AUPMC runs a graduate research programme, and over the last fifteen years thirty students have successfully completed higher degrees, seven, including Amanda Howe (UEA), Moyez Jiwa (Perth) and Gina Higginbottom (Alberta), becoming full professors.

The medical school was reorganised again in 2010 with the formation of five new research departments, none of which have provided a research synergy with general practice. This anomaly has been addressed by putting the AUPMC under the administrative 'umbrella' of medical education so that its identity can be maintained.

In the late 1990s, the University of Sheffield set up the University of Malaya medical school with Professor Mathers and Gary Butler responsible for the general practice component of the Sheffield curriculum. During this time an academic exchange programme was created and a number of joint research studies were completed. Other connections with the Far East include a long-standing research collaboration with Fu-Jen University, Taiwan (Professor Yu Chu Huang), which has resulted in collaborative studies on postnatal depression and cross-cultural health needs assessment in minority populations.

*David Hannay*
*Nigel Mathers*

# Chapter 19

# The University of Southampton

## 1969–1980

Southampton was one of the three new medical schools founded in the wake of the Todd report – the first new school in the UK since before the First World War (as we were constantly reminded). It prided itself on being different and set out to at least double the then very low proportion of clinical teaching in the community (achieving 7 per cent in the first decade). The foundation Dean, the epidemiologist Donald Acheson (later Sir Donald Acheson, CMO at the DHSS), had made his name in Oxford with his record linkage project. He brought with him an able general practitioner from nearby Bicester, John Forbes, who had helped him, particularly with aspects of care of the elderly. Forbes was appointed as senior lecturer in Acheson's department of community medicine in 1968, with the brief of developing general practice education and research and including a model practice. At first medical school money was 'ring fenced' from the other Southampton faculties and further appointments rapidly followed: David Skelton as lecturer in 1969, Chris Metcalfe as senior lecturer in 1970, myself in 1972 and Pat Hertnon from New Zealand in 1973 as lecturers to complete the initial staffing of the university practice.

The Southampton department was thus 'practice based'. Lying near the city boundary, the serendipitous extension of the boundary to form a large new housing estate allowed the practice to grow rapidly without 'poaching' patients from local general practitioners. This encouraged one of John Forbes's greatest achievements – the development of the academic health centre at Aldermoor, initially in a temporary building.

A key feature was research ambition and the flagship project (indeed for many years the only project) was a major scheme to deliver 'age-specific primary care', funded by the Nuffield Foundation for the then fabulous sum of £110,000 over seven years. This set out to test a proposition by another epidemiologist, Tom McKeown, that medicine was now too complex for a single general practitioner to encompass; his answer was to appoint primary care paediatricians, geriatricians and, in between, 'mediatricians'. David Skelton had worked in geriatrics with McKeown in Birmingham, Chris Metcalfe had achieved the paediatric MRCP entirely from his father's practice in Bedford, and I had the adult MRCP and so was one obvious mediatrician. The other, Pat Hertnon, was a charismatic and experienced general practitioner, exactly two metres tall and favouring purple suits. Only John Forbes had any research experience.

John Forbes himself was forceful and energetic and generated impressive support and participation in teaching from general practitioners all over Wessex. The newly independent department of primary medical care split off from community medicine under his leadership, and he was awarded a personal chair. The first forty students arrived in 1971, and general practice 'early medical contact' in year one was a flagship feature. These first students' visits featured afternoon tea on the lawn of doctors' houses in Romsey and Lymington. Five years later the full curriculum was in place with substantial general practice input in first, third and final years and a network of over 100 general practice teachers all over the Wessex region.[1] The age-specific care project was also well launched,[2] supported by an innovative main-frame computer clinical record system in the practice – the brainchild of the charismatic programme director, Ewen Clark, another talented Scot, recruited after three years in Gainesville, Florida. The practice expanded to over 8,000 patients and in 1976 moved into a splendid new permanent building. Clinical accommodation at street level supported academic seminar rooms and offices above, with generous car-parking sited on the direct route between the university campus and the main teaching hospital at Southampton General. In 1972 the department was proud to host the first ASM after formal constitution of the new AUTGP. The meeting was held in idyllic weather in a local Roman Catholic teacher-training college and the department had truly 'arrived'.

Multiple personnel issues limited the department's development between 1976 and 1980. John Forbes retired early due to ill health and his replacement, Nigel Stott, who arrived on New Year's Day 1979 with high hopes all round, found a very messy situation just too hard and decided to resign after only three months in post. This felt like the nadir to those of us remaining, but Nigel had already appointed two very bright new lecturers – David Jewell and George Lewith, the latter now a leading figure in the world of alternative medicine.

*George Freeman*

## 1980–1998

After the inevitable long academic process the chair was re-advertised and the appointment of John Bain in 1980 launched a complete turn around in fortune, based on a strong research programme and several academic appointments, most notably Ann Louise Kinmonth and Roger Jones, but also Charles Freer and Ian Gregg. John was looking for heavyweight general practice research experience – rare at that time. Ian was a Kingston general practitioner who had for some years taken a pioneering role in general practice orientated asthma research at the Brompton Hospital – sufficient to gain him his Oxford DM on the basis of a series of published papers alone. These appointments heralded the growth of a substantial research programme focusing on common and chronic clinical conditions in general practice. Research grants from the MRC, the Nuffield Provincial Hospitals Trust and Wessex Health Authority led to important original work on otitis media, asthma, diabetes, cardiovascular disease and gastro-intestinal disorders. A 'new blood' chair of primary care epidemiology was filled by David Mant and the three Wellcome training fellowships in primary care were won by Simon Griffin, Paul Little and Stephen Morgan. This research was ably supported by a group of dedicated non-medical researchers prominent among whom were Nicki Spiegal, Elizabeth Murphy, Fran Ross, Joan Dunleavy, Sue Lydiard, Lindsey Agius and Sally Richards. An innovative project was developed with the King's Fund which led to management development within the department and courses on leadership became an integral part of ongoing activities in the unit. The undergraduate teaching programme continued to flourish and the fourth-year study in-depth allowed a wide range of students to become an integral part of the research programme. Beyond the confines of the UK, senior staff made important contributions to NAPCRG (the North American Primary Care Research Group).

A formative decade characterised by teaching was thus followed by a research decade which put the department in a favourable position for the first RAE in 1992. During the early 1990s, Roger Jones, John Bain and George Freeman left to fill chairs in Newcastle, Dundee and Charing Cross & Westminster. David Jewell, who had moved to the new department at Bristol, became editor of the *BJGP*. Ann Louise Kinmonth became professor and head of department in 1992, leaving to take the chair in Cambridge in 1996, being followed as head of department by Helen Smith.

## 1998–2010

Tony Kendrick, a mentee of Paul Freeling at St George's, was appointed to the vacant chair and head of department in 1998 and added a new strand of research on mental health problems in primary care. In his first year as head of department he set about separating the practice downstairs from the academic department upstairs. The reasons for this were academic (it was a very peculiar practice with lots of part-time academic general practitioners which didn't provide a representative base for teaching and research), financial (the school of medicine was paying overheads to the central university on more than thirty practice staff it didn't need to employ), and humane (the patients were almost never able to see a doctor without a student present, were always being asked to take part in research studies, and saw too many different doctors coming and going). After the Aldermoor surgery became an ordinary NHS practice, the six academic general practitioners working upstairs were seconded to practices across the region, one in each of the six local primary care groups, helping to spread the influence of the department. So the department became a 'practice-linked' rather than 'practice-based' department, which was by now the model favoured by almost all departments in the UK.

Soon after Tony Kendrick's arrival, David Mant left to take up the chair and headship at Oxford, and Paul Little was awarded the first and only MRC clinician scientist fellowship to be awarded to a general practitioner, which supported the development of his remarkably successful research programme on strategies to reduce antibiotic prescribing for acute infections in general practice. Helen Smith worked extremely hard to develop the Wessex Research Network (WreN), involving hundreds of practices in large-scale clinical trials led by the department, before she was appointed to the first chair of general practice at the new Brighton and Sussex medical school.

The general practice teaching group led by Jenny Field, Chris Stephens and Nick Dunn moved to a different division within Southampton in 2001, taking a leading role in educational developments for the whole medical school (Chris Stephens becoming director of education and Jenny Field director of the four-year graduate entry programme), but effectively now working separately from the research group which remained at Aldermoor.

Following a disappointing result in the 2001 RAE, and the subsequent failure of Southampton's application to join the NIHR school for primary care research in 2004, the group really worked hard to concentrate its research efforts in three strands: acute infections, mental health and complementary therapies (led by George Lewith). This led to a much more successful RAE result in 2008, and subsequent admission to the NIHR school. In 2010, Tony Kendrick left to take up the post of Dean of Hull York medical school.

*George Freeman*
*John Bain*
*Tony Kendrick*

## Notes

1. Metcalfe G.C., Freeman G.K., Bain D.J.G. and Rowe L.J., 'Teaching primary medical care in Southampton: the first decade', *Lancet*, 1, 1983: 697–9.
2. Clark E.M. and Forbes J.A., *Evaluating Primary Care*, London, Croom-Helm, 1979.

# Chapter 20

# The London Medical Schools

In 1967, all London medical schools were separate institutions based on their teaching hospitals, many of which had moved from their original central sites. Successive attempts at merger met resistance, but by 2000 there were just five undergraduate schools, all incorporated in large multi-faculty colleges with the exception of St George's.

## IMPERIAL COLLEGE LONDON

In the north-west, Imperial College absorbed St Mary's Hospital in 1989 and in 1997 also took in Charing Cross and Westminster Hospitals (already merged in 1983).

### Charing Cross Hospital

*Early development of general practice teaching*
Charing Cross Hospital medical school started in the mid-nineteenth century at the hospital building near The Strand, London. It was small, taking twenty to thirty new students annually. General practice teaching started in the 1950s when students were invited to stay with a general practitioner (usually an alumnus) for three weeks in their final year. Most practices were outside London (often rural), enabling students to experience the daily life of a general practitioner, including out of hours work and living with his family.

Charing Cross Hospital moved to Fulham in 1974, and the annual school intake increased to 120. The final-year general practice attachment expanded accordingly and the Dean, Professor Glenister, initiated plans for an undergraduate general practice teaching unit. The education committee of the north and west London faculty of the RCGP took great interest in the developments, especially as the GMC was threatening to remove accreditation from schools that did not have departments of general practice.

In 1977, Colin Leonard was appointed senior lecturer for five sessions per week. Trained in Birmingham, he had practised in a north Cotswold market town for twelve years. He had been active in the RCGP experimental courses study group in London, and in the 1974 RCGP Nuffield training for course organisers, set up by Paul Freeling and Susie Barry. This last stimulated a radical rethink of general practice teaching at all levels. Edward Shaoul, who had developed some local general practice teaching, was appointed honorary senior lecturer.

### Getting started

We decided to take advantage of the final-year attachment as it stood and to preface it with a course in the fourth year, using principles of experiential learning. This two-course programme enabled both the discrete intensification of learning by 'second visiting', a domain well recognised and used in general practice consultations, and the use of experiences themselves as a means of promoting learning rather than each student aiming towards specific objectives at set times – a hope often defeated by the pragmatic nature of general practice in the demand-led service of that time. It also enabled the organisers and teachers to learn by their experience of the courses.

### Recruitment of teachers

General practitioners were sought by invitation and questionnaire sent to all practices within five miles of Charing Cross Hospital in the Ealing, Hammersmith and Hounslow family practitioner committee area. Shaoul already had a list of keen local general practitioners. They offered their time without payment and gave generous support to the development of the department – the good will was remarkable. Meetings were held where details of the proposed course and teaching method were rehearsed and refined. By the time the first course was running there were about fifty local teachers available to host students for four of the five days of the course. 'In house' teaching and group work was undertaken largely by general practice teachers and their practice staff. This demanded much effort in setting the scene, reflection, discussion and feedback from students and teachers alike. To clarify the experimental and idiosyncratic form and method of these courses they were named 'general practice workshops'. We created and adjusted workbooks, and progressively altered our input to introduction and feedback sessions.

In the early 1980s, with the support of Dr (later Professor) Catherine Peckham, a structure of 'hub and spoke' geographically linked groups of general practice teachers was proposed to enable better peer support and allow teaching developments to be implemented locally, with six 'tutors' responsible for a cluster of general practice teachers in their immediate locality. No money was available for these appointments either. The academic unit of general practice had no fixed office, but depended on help from secretaries from supportive departments, medical school administration, and Colin Leonard's practice. There was a requirement to publish research attached to the senior lecturer post, however there was no support to enable this to happen. The research that was done was largely collaborative and in continuing medical education – the Educational Research Project funded by the DHSS and run at the RCGP during 1979–1988 being the best-known example.

## Westminster Hospital

Westminster was slower to get started, but in 1975 James Scobie, a general practitioner in Barnes, was appointed part-time senior lecturer on condition that he took the MRCGP examination (which he duly passed). He set up a network of a dozen practices taking students for (unpaid) two-week attachments supported by seminars and staff development meetings. However, general practice was located in an unsympathetic department of community medicine, and eventually James was dismissed after the medical school, in his words, 'lost patience with me. The Dean told me that one of the complaints about me was that I had sought advice from David Morrell at St Thomas's!'

In the wider campus, following the 1983 merger to make Charing Cross and Westminster Medical School, the academic general practice unit was briefly given space at St Stephen's Hospital Chelsea, though this was shortly to be demolished to make way for the new Chelsea and Westminster Hospital. Most teachers who had taught Westminster students became available again. James Scobie was recruited once more, together with Bruce Armstrong, Alwyn Latham, Mel Henry, Graham Cassels Brown and Geoffrey Dove.

In 1985 the unit came under Professor Ariel Lant in the department of clinical pharmacology and therapeutics. He enabled the hub and spoke 'cluster groups' to be firmly reinforced and their nine leaders (eventually Bruce Armstrong, Grant Blair, Rimah El-Borai, David Filer, Stephen Hirst, Jenny Lebus, Alastair Mitchell, Ed Shaoul and Adam Snape) to be funded. The now regular meetings with tutors provided a useful communication mechanism between the teaching general practitioners and the school.

### Second merger

By the early 1990s, preparations were being made to combine with St Mary's to form the Imperial College Faculty of Medicine. In 1993, George Freeman was appointed professor of general practice. New appointments included Mary Pierce, Jon Fuller and Jim Kennedy and a full-time teaching administrator, Caroline Goodman. The availability of SIFT money, combined with the London Implementation Zone Educational Initiatives (LIZEI) programme, enabled Charing Cross and Westminster to be a credible and substantial partner in this merger. All but one of the former 'tutors' were appointed again in their enhanced role as academic facilitators, fully funded at one clinical session per week at honorary consultant rates, initiating a very considerable increase in the amount and quality of teaching in primary care.

The two departments finally united on one site in 2000 in the refurbished medical school building at Charing Cross hospital in Fulham, led by Brian Hurwitz, and joining with the department of social medicine led by Professor Gerry Stimson.

*Colin Leonard*
*George Freeman*
*James Scobie*

### St Mary's Hospital

In the early 1950s Geoffrey Barber had invited groups of Mary's students to visit him for a day to get a taste of general practice, and in the 1960s, Harry Levitt, a former chairman of the RCGP, unsuccessfully attempted to set up a department at St Mary's. However, early in 1971, St Mary's Hospital medical school obtained funding from the DHSS and advertised for a part-time tutor in general practice. Marshall Marinker was appointed and placed in Geoffrey Rose's department of epidemiology and preventive medicine.

**Marshall Marinker** writes: 'The department was situated in the old railway stables adjacent to Paddington station. The seminar room placed at my disposal had once accommodated the dray horses! It was windowless and ventilated by a system of conduits from a nearby pharmacological laboratory, so that every now and then we would be flooded with pungent clouds of chemical solvent. Yet I could not have been happier, and none could have been more welcoming, helpful, understanding and supportive than so many of the senior staff at Mary's.' His two-week teaching slot in the second clinical year was based on a secondment to a teaching practice; the clinical tutors included Harry Levitt, Bill Styles (secretary of College council), his partner Stuart Carne (College treasurer and later president) and Lotte Newman (also later College president). The secondments focused on problem solving, probability, communication and ethical challenges.

When, a year later, he was appointed senior lecturer, Marshall reported: 'The Dean was beside himself as I asked for yet more time – a third week. The Dean said "Does Marshall not realise that, as we speak, every single student spends two whole weeks on his course, while only half of the students are able to attend the course on cardiovascular surgery?"'

Things were not much different when **Conrad Harris** arrived in 1974. He writes: 'My first morning at St Mary's was memorable. I asked the School Secretary where my new department was and when I could advertise for a secretary. He looked nonplussed, and told me that no-one had imagined that I would want either a room or a secretary, but he would think about it. Worse was to come: when I went to the dining room for lunch, the professor of medicine came up to me and said "I hope you realise that if I hadn't been away on the day, there would never have been a decision to have a department of general practice." The only time he ever spoke to me again was a few months later. "Tell me one thing you can teach that I don't already teach." "How about ante-natal care?" He didn't pursue the subject. The rest of the teaching staff were not like this – though they were a little bemused at the idea that a northern general practitioner might be able to do anything useful for St Mary's; Geoffrey Rose was always a friend.

The only space available was not a room but a length of corridor with shelves of pathology specimens on both sides, frequently inspected by students; it had swing doors at each end. Refusing this marked me out as a difficult customer. Eventually I found a derelict prefabricated hut by the side of the canal, and this became the new department. The other basic requirement of the job was a practice for my clinical work – I was very happy in the one that I found in Fulham (where, later, George Freeman also worked for fifteen years).

Turning to more academic matters, the first need was to appoint many more teaching practices, both local and regional. Next came a vocational training scheme, which brought with it a relationship with a London deanery, as well as organising the day release course. Increasing work needed more staff; over time I was able to recruit Patrick Pietroni,

Paul Wallace and Andy Haines, while Brian Jarman was given another two sessions for research. In 1978 we left the canal to go to the new Lisson Grove Health Centre.

I'd been pondering the idea of a pre-registration year that included four months each of medicine, surgery and general practice – a revolutionary idea at the time. I started talking to various St Mary's consultants who were already involved in pre-registration education and training. There was not much interest, but the professor of surgery was willing to take part, and Brian Jarman offered his practice. It was harder to get a medical post, but when one appeared I floated the idea at Mary's. There were no strong views either way, and I was advised to approach the Medical Board of London University.

After a rather lonely four-year battle (for three years I had no support at all), help duly appeared from an unlikely quarter. Dame Sheila Sherlock, the renowned liver specialist and a hard-line opponent of my proposal, was put on the sub-committee charged with bringing the matter to a conclusion. She ended her comments by saying "I know in my heart that this is wrong", but her fervour had the effect of moving members in the opposite direction; the Board later ratified the experiment. It had been a long battle, but the rotation proved to be a great success. Within a year it was taken up by the Department of Health and it was soon rolled out nationally.

The next important event was money offered to St Mary's for a Chair, which was given to Brian Jarman in 1984. I moved to Leeds in 1986.'

Brian Jarman became full-time professor in January 1984 and Andy Haines – senior partner in a group practice in Craven Park Health Centre in Harlesden, who also worked part-time for the MRC epidemiology and medical care unit – was appointed to a part-time senior lectureship at the same time. Later Julian Tudor-Hart, Steve Gillam, Paul Wallace and Brian Hurwitz were also appointed as part-time senior lecturers for different periods.

By 1993 the department had moved back to the former Grand Union Canal warehouses in South Wharf Road. After joining with Charing Cross and Westminster, Brian Jarman was appointed as head of the merged department, being replaced at his retirement in 1998 by Brian Hurwitz. The two wings of the enlarged department finally co-located in fine refurbished accommodation on the Charing Cross site.

*Marshall Marinker*
*Conrad Harris*
*Andy Haines*
*Brian Jarman*

# KING'S COLLEGE LONDON SCHOOL OF MEDICINE

In 1982, Guy's Hospital Medical School merged with St Thomas's Hospital Medical School to become UMDS (the United Medical and Dental Schools) and then in 1998 with King's to become GKT (Guy's, King's and Thomas's). Since 2005, the combined school has been known as King's College London School of Medicine.

## Guy's Hospital

In the early 1960s, John Butterfield, professor of experimental medicine at Guy's, became involved in a community study of diabetes in Bedford. This sensitised him to the need to introduce general practice teaching at Guy's. In 1963 he met up with Robert Smith, who he had known in the RAMC in the late 1940s as a fellow medical officer in Germany.

**Robert Smith** takes up the story: 'In 1952 I started a general practice in the village of Stanwell, west Middlesex. With the help of William Pickles, John Fry and John Horder, I began research in 1953, studying pain sensitivity in general practice and getting an MD from Trinity College Dublin in 1956. As a result I was offered a part-time appointment on the clinical research staff at the Wellcome Foundation which enabled me to continue with my practice and further my research.

My boss, immunologist Jock Adamson, wanted me to retain a link with his team, thinking it was valuable to have a "real" doctor on board. He asked me "What would you really like to do?" I did not hesitate, "I would like to establish a general practice teaching and research unit in a London medical school." Jock persuaded Wellcome to provide funds for three years, provided I acted as a general practice consultant on pain problems.

Reading the *Evening Standard* in a crowded tube, I spotted a headline "New Town at Woolwich". I suggested to Professor Butterfield that I should apply for the position of physician to the new town to start a teaching practice twelve miles down-river from Guy's. I then visited the Dean at Guy's who, on John's recommendation, was pleased to have his school linked with the new town, soon to be called Thamesmead, the prospect of a new patient population being referred to Guy's being very appealing. John Butterfield asked me "Do you have any money?" When I responded "Yes", he answered, "You can start on Monday!" And so academic general practice began at Guy's.

There were many problems. Clinical space was not available to develop a practice and local doctors were not enthusiastic about joining a Guy's enterprise (nor were Guy's too happy about being involved with them). I had met Sir George Godber, CMO of the NHS, on several occasions. He also was an admirer of Professor Butterfield. He was delighted to hear that Guy's Hospital had become interested in an academic general practice unit. If Guy's were truly interested the job at the new town was mine. So now the development of the new practice site as part of Thamesmead began.

I was co-opted to the Greater London Council (GLC) planning committee to start work on the first practice site. I recruited Michael Curwen to assist in developing the general practice plan, and liaised with the College of General Practitioners and with Guy's in developing a general practice medical student curriculum. In this critical early phase Professor Butterfield helped keep our project afloat in the complex environment of an ancient London medical school. Our funds were inadequate for the task, but with the professor's help we succeeded in obtaining additional funds from the Nuffield Foundation. Our embryonic department was known as the general practice teaching and research unit (GPRU). Some of Guy's diehard administrators initially objected to our small group having any title!

We began volunteer general practice seminars for students in our backstreet office behind Guy's, and arranged visits to surgeries of general practice friends in the London area. I attended in-patient rounds led by Professor Butterfield who kindly drew me into case discussions. John was an ardent cricketer and captain of the hospital team. I played opening bat and made some inroads of acceptance into the Guy's community! We constructed a detailed plan of the town's surgeries, including links with the local hospitals and with other health and welfare services, and outlined the teaching and research to be undertaken. Co-ordinated administration and funding which then had the blessing of all agencies involved was put in place. Details were published in the *Lancet*.[1]

Our plans met a severe blow when major funding cuts to the NHS began in 1965. The GPRU at the bottom of the totem pole at Guy's had little hope for its future plans. The only funds that were certain were what I could earn as a general practitioner at Thamesmead. In 1968, I accepted an appointment as professor at the University of North Carolina, Chapel Hill. My successor, Peter Higgins, is to be admired for having taken control of what then was a sinking ship and continuing until financial matters eventually improved and the GPRU became a fully fledged department at Guy's with its practice base at Thamesmead.'

**Donald Craig**, one of the members of the department, continues the story: 'The department of general practice at Guy's emerged as three movements coincided. The GLC was to build a huge new town on the Erith Marsh. Guy's Hospital had a mind to follow its Deptford patients and to instigate an integrated health service there. Experiments and innovations in student teaching, with an emphasis on epidemiology and early exposure to real-life patients were becoming fashionable.

Peter Higgins arrived in 1968 followed by Rodney Turner in 1970. They practised from portakabins and later from Lakeside Health Centre. This elegant building housed dental services and a full panoply of medical and social co-workers. Peripheral consultant clinics were instituted in a wide range of specialities. However, it was always diffi-cult to provide a satisfactory cohort for the given specialist on the given day.

Lakeside was to be a permanent but peripheral health centre until the main development arrived. During this period of inter-disciplinary wrangling the department had the unvarying support of Bob Rigg (GLC Thamesmead architect) and Derek Stow (architect of both health centres). Gallions Reach Health Centre was erected after many vicissi-tudes in the early 1980s. I assisted in its realisation – perhaps the largest health centre of its time. Meantime we inhabited flats, conjoined houses, and extravagant pre-fabs. The final building incorporated an in-house pharmacy and a whole floor devoted to expected developments of the department. The growth of the estate had to be mirrored in partnership expansion. There was constant conflict between the service role and the desire to institute research. Protected time was not available.

The Bernard Sunley professorship was instituted in the early 1970s thereby establishing a formal department. Its finances were always shrouded in mystery extending to the presence of an *eminence grise*, Michael Curwen. Skirmishes occurred as each new partner endeavoured to obtain a 'departmental session'. These were seen as a necessary acco-lade and were highly valued.

The sense of isolation experienced by the patients – removed from the support of Deptford – was mirrored in the health centres, and efforts were made to nourish group morale among the staff. A community workers' group encompassing all workers on Thamesmead met weekly. The local team of priests played a prominent part in each surgery, inter-ceding in staff difficulties, and one usually accompanied us as a process observer on retreats.

Student teaching was ahead of its time and probably unacceptable by today's standards. Clinical students saw patients at first contact on their own. They were expected to elicit the real problem, and suggest a plan and prescription to their supervising doctor. Pre-clinical students experienced real-life interviews. They, three at a time, were introduced to patients who they interviewed in series, and in turn watched their colleagues in action. Different material was invariably produced. There followed a discussion which the patient usually led. David Armstrong (social medicine) and John Weinman (psychology) were participating mentors at that time. Students found the experience stressful but wanted it repeated. Some of these experiences headed the annual Guy's student audit as valuable and exciting.

The professor had an RHA role and instituted both a local vocational course and an evening class (based on peer learning) for middle-aged doctors. The Thamesmead Inter-disciplinary Project (King's Fund) explored the usefulness of educating medical students, health visitors and social workers in parallel for a semester. Findings centred on questions of status, differing expectations, subtleties of language and the degree of supervision expected.

Most of our work was on the Marsh. Very few seminars took place in Guy's despite good fellow-feeling from the consultants. Membership of the AUTGP revealed encouraging progress elsewhere – albeit somewhat conformist by our standards. The Sunley money ran out as the Guy's department was subsumed under the St Thomas's department in 1982. Subsequent developments there seem rather tame by comparison with those uninhibited, heady days of innovation.'

## Reference

Smith R., Curwen M.P., Chamberlain J. and Butterfield W.J.H., 'The Woolwich and Erith project', *Lancet*, i, 1966: 650–4.

## King's College Hospital

When I retired in 2004, my last lecture at King's College was to 1,400 students from eight separate health care courses in four lecture rooms with closed circuit connection – the consequence of the union of the three ancient medical schools of Guy's, St Thomas's and King's. It was a far cry from the one-to-one relationship of general practitioner and trainee that had inspired us in the mid-1970s to take the training agenda into the student curriculum, but the success of this overall venture was such that, by the time of the final merger of these schools at the end of the century, a sixth of the total (clinical and pre-clinical) curriculum in this vast medical school was taught by general practice (under Anne Stephenson's leadership). And the teaching in the practices throughout south London was funded by SIFT on a clear and egalitarian model that our (disgruntled) colleagues in hospitals were not able to demolish.

But such a falsely triumphalist selective memory conceals the almost total lack of support offered by the schools in the early days, and the Byzantine local politics in an area where three departments manoeuvred in one Region and one FHSA. It sometimes seemed as if the clinical struggle in the Walworth Road with drug addicts, crime and poverty was nothing compared to the street-fighting in the school where, as a friend once remarked, 'the battles are so bitter because the stakes are so low'. But we loved (almost) every minute of it.

My general practice trainer John McEwan had developed a brilliant and successful parallel life at King's College Hospital as a national leader in family planning, and it was to him that the school turned when, as the last of the three (alongside St Thomas's and Guy's), King's decided it needed a general practice presence. He had arranged in 1976 for three of us general practitioners to conduct ward teaching, and when in 1978 a five session lectureship was offered, although a single-hander at the time I was lucky enough to be appointed. This enabled me to develop John's cadre of practice teachers, expand my own practice and let John retire back to family planning. In a series of local meetings and weekends at Cambridge colleges, the group of general practitioner teachers united in the sort of comradeship that exclusion builds and developed a new curriculum. It proved so popular with students that when in the late 1980s the hospital was threatened by ward closures and with being unable to deliver its teaching, we took over a 'medical firm' and ran it in local practices under Jeremy Gray and then Paul Booton. The students learned faster than on the wards, with organised and detailed sessions on familiar convalescent patients with defined conditions. Feedback was enthusiastic (occasionally devastating in its comparative – 'at least you turn up...'), so the experiment continued into the mainstream. But we failed to publish the results properly – my own fault, and the department's Achilles' heel.

Because, in contrast to other schools, we did not establish a department practice, the department had a strong central group in portakabins at Denmark Hill. General practice teaching was led initially by Jane Dammers, chronic illness research by Patrick White, and I developed the medical ethics programme. At the time this last was an innovation. I had also been part of a small national group that had set up the *Journal of Medical Ethics*, and currently chair its editorial board.

Two other innovations sprang from a successful series of educational forums. The 'Meet the department' series – brainchild of our young department secretary Jan Prior and the King's casualty consultant,

Ed Glucksman – were monthly meetings between up to a hundred local general practitioners and an individual clinical department from the hospital (in rotation). Departments were asked to bring all their staff and make a presentation over an evening dinner (drug company funded), after which there was an open and frank discussion with the general practitioners present. From this base, Ed and I went on to set up a project in A&E, the hypothesis tested being that patients there could be triaged into either 'real' A&E or primary care problems, and that the latter would be better managed by doctors trained in primary care. The project was brilliantly run by Jeremy Dale, and the results were conclusive: the general practitioners more than halved investigations, prescribing and admissions while maintaining good care and patient satisfaction. The idea was rolled out locally and nationally, and Jeremy became professor at Warwick.

Another innovation arose from the dissatisfaction often voiced about standards and services across the primary/secondary care interface. I had been chair (1977–1985) of a group who had campaigned for, designed and built probably the first UK intermediate care centre, a sort of 'cottage hospital come to town' close to St Thomas's. Initially every political and medical group was in opposition except the community health council, but it gained national acceptance (after being opened by Charles and Diana, with an MBE for the chair) and patient enthusiasm. Our first AIDS patient was looked after and died there. The success did not endear us with St Thomas's, who had opposed the centre. But this work established the King's department with a third 'arm' – that of primary care development. An inspired and intensely hard working team led by Virginia Morley and Tyrrell Evans, backed by King's Fund money amongst other funding, toured local practices to discover their needs and set up individual and group responses to issues as various as clinical waste, hospital timetables and diabetes shared care. The FHSA were of the opinion that this project was a major factor in the improvements in local general practices observed from the 1980s on, and later funded our first proper departmental premises by giving us an extra floor of a new build at Denmark Hill. Later still they asked us to take on the management of a failing local practice (now a local leader). But we did not reckon with the power of the RAE (which rejected medical ethics) or the need for a merger, which took us finally and happily into bed with St Thomas's and Guy's and off the Denmark Hill site.

We were lucky, as latecomers, to be inspired by the first wave of general practice teachers and academics and to be working in what seems now to have been a golden age of general practice with wide and enthusiastic support from a large number of local primary care clinicians. We were lucky too to be able to make links, inside the hospital and out, with colleagues with whom we clicked, and to be able to fish in every financial pool we could think of. And we were lucky to be supported by an FHSA for whom we were something of a Godsend, and to be young with supportive practices and families. A lot of it was chaotic. We got too large, with all sorts of add-ons like audit, nursing development, telephone advice training and so on; we seldom said 'no' a new project; we spent a lot of time in group reflection and away days resolving conflicts; and we did not subject our work rigorously enough to the searchlight of research. But it was fun, and, who knows, someone somewhere might have benefited.

*Roger Higgs*


## St Thomas's Hospital

### Early years

The development of academic general practice in London in 1967 was slow because many members of the consultant staff in the teaching hospitals regarded the quality of general practitioner care in their immediate vicinity as inadequate and were not prepared to expose their students to medicine in the community. This was not entirely unjustified as general practice in the city was very variable, some of it excellent but a good deal exceptionally poor. It was therefore incumbent on any academic developing a department to demonstrate that high quality clinical care could be provided in this setting. For this reason some departments developing in London were based on practices where this could be demonstrated.

At St Thomas's, a senior lectureship in general practice was established in 1967 in the department of clinical epidemiology headed by Professor Walter Holland. The post was funded by a research grant from the DH through Sir George Godber, the CMO. The appointment was for three years, during which the person appointed was required to demonstrate, by research, the difference between medicine practised in hospital and in general practice. The practice to be involved was selected by Lord Stephen Taylor, a governor at St Thomas's, based on a survey he had carried out prior to publishing his book *Good General Practice*. He chose the practice of George Gage, situated half a mile from the hospital and providing care for 5,000 patients. David Morrell, who had worked for three years with Richard Scott in Edinburgh, was appointed to the post. He was told to spend six elevenths of his time providing clinical care in the practice and the remainder developing research.

In anticipation of this appointment, Lord Taylor and the Dean of the medical school had persuaded the Lambeth Council to build a group practice centre where Dr Gage's practice could unite with another local practice. Situated within a mile of St Thomas's, this was designed to be the new teaching and research centre for general practice for the medical school. After four years in 'shop front premises', this union came in 1971, providing care for 10,000 patients. Bill Marson and Luke Zander joined the project. For the first time in Lambeth, community nurses and health visitors were attached to the practice. Thanks to the quality and dedication of the doctors appointed, the practice quickly acquired a reputation for providing high quality medical care. In 1972 the department of general practice was established. Gage was appointed as a part-time senior lecturer and Marson and Zander as senior lecturers. Shortly afterwards, Chris Watkins was appointed as a lecturer.

Between 1969 and 1971 four papers were published in refereed medical journals describing the difference between medicine practised in hospital and in the community. Sir George Godber was delighted with this work and, with Sir Keith Joseph, approached the Wolfson Foundation to endow the first department of general practice in the University of London. In 1974 David Morrell was appointed Wolfson professor of general practice.

Undergraduate teaching played a small part in the work of the department in its early years when it was fully occupied in developing the clinical base and its research. From 1969 onwards, however, clinical attachments to local general practices were established, and a new half-day release course for trainees was developed. At the beginning of the next decade, with help from John Wynn Owen, the chief executive at St Thomas's, a full rotating trainee programme was established based on the teaching hospital and directed by Michael Courtenay.

By the 1980s the department was expanding but was constrained by lack of finance. It depended entirely on the income of the practice, the DHSS research grant and the good will of local general practitioners. During a period of inflation the Wolfson endowment was reinvested to provide some security for the future but it was not then available to the developing department. In spite of this the department was producing numerous research papers, often in association with the social scientists, epidemiologists and statisticians in the Health Service Research Unit. A fellowship course for local general practitioners was developed with support from the St Thomas's Special Trustees. At the instigation of Professor Higgins at Guy's, this later became the first MSc in general practice in the University of London. Undergraduate education was extended into the pre-clinical years and proper clerkships in general practice were established. Courses in communication skills, sexual problems in medicine and medical ethics were developed in association with the departments of psychiatry and obstetrics. The head of department was elected sub-Dean at St Thomas's, and when in 1982 Guy's and St Thomas's were amalgamated, he became chairman of the education committee of the United Medical and Dental Schools (UMDS).

In clinical care the department developed and measured the outcome of integrated ante-natal care with the department of obstetrics, and community diabetic care with the department of endocrinology. High-quality recruitment to the department occurred in the 1980s with the appointment of Martin Roland, Debbie Sharp and Fiona Ross, all of whom went on to develop their own departments. The headship of the department was handed over to Professor Roger Jones in 1994.

### The second generation

Development and expansion then took place against the background of major organisational changes in the NHS and the medical schools. The LIZEI funding, aimed at improving general practitioner recruitment in London, allowed the establishment of new posts related to medical education and the creation of the first primary care skills centre on the site of the old Lambeth Walk group practice in the tower block on Kennington Road. With generous support from the Special Trustees of Guy's and St Thomas's we refurbished the art deco Lambeth Baths building, providing state-of-the-art facilities for the practice, for teaching and for an expanding research group, who had very considerable research support from the Lambeth and Southwark FHSA. This was the era of our successful national negotiations to get some of the SIFT funding out of hospitals and into general practice and of the equally successful campaign to obtain better NHS R&D and MRC funding to support primary care research. We recruited new academic staff, and have been pleased to see Nicky Britten, John Campbell, Jane Ogden, Peter Cantillon and Val Wass go on to chairs and leadership positions elsewhere in the university system. Research flourished and the department had a high profile in fields such as concordance, gastrointestinal disorders, health psychology and patient access and satisfaction.

Two other initiatives in the late 1990s acted as models for major academic developments in later years. The London Academic Trainee Scheme (LATS), funded by LIZEI, allowed general practice trainees to extend their training by spending a year in an academic department and to use this as a springboard to an academic career. This idea has been widely adopted as part of an academic career structure for general practice. The second was the establishment of StaRNeT, the south Thames primary care research network, generously funded at regional level and involving a swathe of practices across the south-east of England. StaRNeT provided the model for many future networks and our experiences helped shape today's UK Primary Care Research Network.

Our Masters programme in general practice continued to flourish and played a significant role in working with the NHS to make careers in general practice more attractive and also to assist in the induction of EU doctors working in London. The Centre for Caribbean Health was located within the department, stimulating training and research related to the large Caribbean population in south-east London. The financial realities of general practice gradually rendered our practice-based departmental model unsustainable, and the Lambeth Walk group practice evolved into a separate NHS organisation, while retaining close teaching and research links with the department.

Key events in the next few years included the amalgamation of the King's College Hospital Medical School department with UMDS on the Lambeth site, as part of GKT – the Guy's, King's and St Thomas's School of Medicine, now with responsibility for about 15 per cent of the undergraduate curriculum, and with an annual student intake of well over 400. In 2005 GKT was re-titled the King's College London School of Medicine and finally, returning to at least some of our roots, we created a joint department of primary care and public health sciences in common accommodation on the Guy's site.

*David Morrell*
*Roger Jones*

## QUEEN MARY COLLEGE

Two more London teaching hospitals with long histories remain on their original sites – Bart's within the old City and the London just in the East End. Long-term pressure from the University of London for amalgamation was strenuously resisted, mutual suspicion extending to the local general practitioners. Eventually, rationalisation under Queen Mary College with relocation of the joint general practice department to the main Whitechapel campus took place in 1995.

### St Bartholomew's Hospital

In 1974 I jumped off *Lord Moran's* Ladder to join Mal Salkind in a lock-up shop practice in Well Street, Hackney. I was the only principal under forty in Hackney, which was officially deemed over-doctored. When Mal, who ran the local vocational training scheme (VTS), was appointed adviser in general practice to Bart's, it became legitimate for two of us to share the VTS work with caring for his 2,800 patients.

A year later Reggie Shooter, the Dean at Bart's, asked Mal to establish a general practice teaching unit that would take the 120 fourth-year undergraduate students for a month – to include at least two weeks attached individually to practices. He promised unusually generous financial support for travel, board and lodging anywhere in the country. Mal appointed an initial core of me, Jimmy Carne and Jack Norrell, who had been with him in the London Teachers' Workshop. I had just embarked on Nuffield III course[1] and was passionately committed to teaching, this dictating a focus on teaching rather than research. Reggie Shooter provided rooms in the old science block in Charterhouse Square.

By 1978 we had developed a general practice curriculum centred on a behavioural model relating to why patients consult their doctors. We started with an initial orientation at Bart's, then two weeks individual attachment in general practice, half inside London and half living-in with practices as far afield as the Isle of Lewis. The final week was back at Bart's for students to share experiences and report on their practice projects.

Our first firm, a very engaged Oxbridge group, didn't mince their words at evaluation. They found hanging around Bart's for a week before moving into proper general practice intolerable. So we telescoped the introduction into the first half of the week, giving extra time in practice. With a curriculum in place and three core teaching practices we felt we had made a start.

Later in 1979 Lesley Southgate returned from London Ontario with her MClinSci. She was appointed a full-time lecturer, with a part-time clinical attachment at Well Street. Jon Fuller, fresh from Bart's and the Hackney VTS, joined Lower Clapton Health Centre, where local general practitioners had been reluctant to move (save my first trainee David Sloan). It had ample consulting and teaching space. Ernie Cooke, an established Hackney general practitioner, was also appointed. His interests included in-patient varicose ulcer treatment at Bethnal Green Hospital. When this closed he used his interest in micro-circulation to set up the thermography unit at Bart's. Ernie broadened our academic focus and we started some research into chlamydia in the community. When Mal got funding to develop computers in general practice, Well Street got its first – the size of a fridge in its own air-conditioned cupboard.

Computer program development remained an important departmental focus, producing the GP Care program, used by several local practices and a handful of practices nationally until the late 1990s.

After the 1982 Black Report,[2] we approached the London deanery about 'The Inner-City Lectureships' scheme – intended for bright young graduates from the local VTS. They were to work half time in local practices and half time at Bart's. In 1983 Sam Heard, an Australian from the Hackney VTS, joined single-hander Gerald Lawson – just turned sixty, reclusive, dedicated to his patients but struggling. This sadly brief partnership ended with Gerald's death eighteen months later. Now the Lawson Practice, they moved to the renovated basement of St Leonards Hospital – a successful example to others. When Sam became principal the vacant lectureship became available and in 1985 Jonathan Graffy joined him from Leicester.

In 1983 the London Hospital finally agreed to an academic general practice department, but we offered them little help at first. However, following the Acheson Report[3] in 1981, funding for two new London general practice chairs became available. If the departments at Bart's and the London merged they would be awarded half the money. So they did in 1984 and funding became available for Brian Harris and Sally Hull from the London, plus four HEFC funded posts including Mal Salkind (professor), Lesley Southgate (senior lecturer) and another of my trainees, Peter Toon, as lecturer. Our accommodation at Charterhouse Square grew by 60 per cent.

The first appointment in the new joint department was innovative and strengthened the relationship between the two schools. Having done sessions in St Botolph's crypt, Peter Toon thought the department should get involved in the community around the London. He proposed a general practice lecturer to work with the homeless. This was approved by the DH and John Collins was appointed, consulting in premises in St Botolph's. This was not an established practice so he was given special permission for his own prescription pads. As I recall, this permission was negotiated by an Act of Parliament.

*Paul Julian*

**Gene Feder** continues: 'In 1988, I came to Bart's as a part-time research fellow to research the health and care of Traveller Gypsies. Research was not Mal Salkind's priority, but he agreed to an application (successful) to the north Thames locally organised research scheme (LORS), a source of HSR funding crucial to fledgling primary care research in east London. In 1990, Lesley Southgate succeeded Mal, bringing a commitment to research and local practice development. Under her watch, the

Bart's and London departments joined together happily, years before the shotgun wedding of the two medical schools.

Synergy between research and development, one of the hallmarks of the joint department, was exemplified by the City and Hackney clinical guidelines programme, and the 'Healthy Eastenders' project, led by John Robson, Kambiz Boomla and Sally Hull, became a national leader in primary care quality improvement through practice level audit and guidance on primary prevention and chronic disease management. Engagement with local practices enabled a series of cluster randomised trials on the management of chronic conditions, such as diabetes, coronary heart disease and asthma. These robust, high-profile studies were led by me and Chris Griffiths, another Hackney general practitioner, and represented our department's coming of age in research.

From 1992, our move to the forefront of primary care trial methodology was largely thanks to our statistician, Sandra Eldridge. Yvonne Carter became our leader in 1995, securing more HEFC funded posts from the medical school and building closer collaborations with primary care groups, as well as encouraging researchers to bid more ambitiously for external funding. Chris and I were joined by Martin Underwood and Stefanie Taylor, who developed programmes in musculoskeletal health and chronic respiratory disease respectively. I developed the first UK research programme on primary care domestic violence, and Chris's respiratory research became nationally and internationally recognised. In the 1990s we embraced qualitative research and systematic reviews, particularly on ethnic minorities and inequality.

Yvonne moved to Warwick in 2004, and Martin became head of the department, now named the centre for health science research. In the 2008 RAE, the department was ranked fourth nationally in HSR. That year Martin passed the reins on to Chris, Sandra followed Yvonne to Warwick, and I moved to Bristol.'

## The London Hospital

The department of general practice at the London Hospital, Whitechapel, only began in the 1980s. General practice in east London, indeed in most of London, still went under the shadow of the 1950 Collings Report.[4] The Dean, Professor Sir John Ellis – an expert on medical education – had a very poor opinion of local general practice, but arranged short residential attachments for the students in suburban and rural practices run by general practitioners who were London Hospital alumni.

In 1981 the Acheson Report stimulated the start of a change at the

London. Brian Harris (Jubilee St Practice, Stepney) was one of four general practitioner members on the Report committee. Four of the 114 recommendations referred to the importance of London teaching hospitals developing academic departments of general practice, and fostering primary care in the areas they served. This resulted in a grant from the north-east Thames RHA to the London Hospital Medical College to create a general practice academic unit. Also funded was the 'Centre for the Study of Primary Care' in Steels Lane Health Centre, Stepney (with the Jubilee St Practice). Brian Harris was medical director of this unit for its lifetime (approximately 1986–1995).

I started as a partner in the Jubilee St Practice in 1980, having trained at St Thomas's. Initially I built links with the London Hospital by taking a post as clinical assistant in rheumatology. As I wanted to teach general practice I started discussions with Eva Alberman, professor of clinical epidemiology, who was very supportive of the need for a department.

In 1981 John Ellis stepped down as Dean due to illness, and Professor Mike Floyer became acting Dean. Initiatives to set up the new department followed promptly. In December 1982 I was summoned along with Brian Harris to interview by David Morrell and Mal Salkind. The London Hospital required that the chosen practice was 'well developed' and had enough space to host medical student teaching on site, so really there was no competition since at the time we were the only practice in Tower Hamlets to be located in a spacious and newly renovated health centre.

Brian was given two senior lecturer sessions and I was offered three as lecturer. This, in the words of my appointment letter, 'left us a little money for the provision of secretarial assistance'. The job description stated that a joint department with Bart's might be established at a later date.

After a most enjoyable first three months in my new post travelling the country and visiting well-established departments such as Southampton and Edinburgh to collect ideas about curriculum development and teaching methods, we opened shop in April 1983, teaching nine firms a year, each lasting one month (week one introduction, weeks two to three peripheral attachment, and week four feedback).

From the start we taught about the consultation, and recruited Mary Burd, a primary care psychologist, to help us. Our course involved video training in consultation skills (using rather primitive video cameras), and a prototype OSCE, and all students ran a group project during their peripheral attachment on subjects such as 'terminal care in general practice', 'do general practitioners practice prevention?' and other classic general practice topics. The teaching was well received, and we recruited a number of Tower Hamlets practices to balance the existing rural exposure. However, due to our skeleton staffing and the weight of teaching responsibilities we were not able to develop research.

In 1984 Mal Salkind was appointed as head of a joint Bart's and the London department of general practice. For some years the teaching continued as before, with Bart's students being taught from Well St Practice and the London students based at Jubilee St Practice, with the clinical teachers meeting to share ideas. The annual tutors' days were initially a bit tense as the general practice tutors, who had strong hospital loyalties, found it difficult to accept the necessity of a combined department.

From around 1988, the two departments integrated progressively with new appointments being made to the joint department, but the process of amalgamation was not fully completed until 1994 when Bart's and the London integrated with Queen Mary, University of London, and moved to its new premises on the Queen Mary campus in 1995.

*Sally Hull*

## Notes

1. Nuffield Course Organisers courses I, II & III; P. Freeling, FRCGP, and Susie M.K. Barry, BSc; six one-week modules run over one year (1974 to 1976).
2. Department of Health and Social Services, *Inequalities in Health*: *Report of a Research Working Group*, London, DHSS, 1980 (the Black Report).
3. London Health Planning Consortium, Primary Health Care Study Group, *Primary Health Care in Inner London*, London, DHSS, 1981 (the Acheson Report).
4. Collings J.S., 'General practice in England today: a reconnaissance', *Lancet*, i, 1950: 55–85.

## ST GEORGE'S HOSPITAL

*Solo beginning within epidemiology and social medicine*

An academic general practice unit started at St George's in 1978, as part of Professor Ted Bennett's department of clinical epidemiology and social medicine, which was housed in a portakabin near what is now the Robert Lowe sports centre. Paul Freeling was the only member of the unit, but in due course he recruited four local general practitioners, Lydia Smythe, Ralph Burton, Richard Chegwidden and Clifford Floyd (also known as the gang of four) to help him develop a teaching programme for undergraduates. St George's at that time provided a single

MBBS course for an approximate intake of 130 students. The 1976 curriculum was horizontally and vertically integrated, and was revolutionary in its day, but had no time allocated to general practice. Paul fought for the time, and was eventually granted ten Tuesday afternoons as part of a ten-week neurology block! Eventually this was consolidated into a two-week attachment to local practices in the third or fourth year, and a great triumph followed with the approval of a four-week attachment for final-year students. Ralph Burton led on this, and developed the links that established our outer ring of teaching practices, with the hubs run by local organisers.

### Sub-department
The now sub-department of general practice moved with clinical epidemiology and social medicine into Jenner Wing. Paul Freeling began to establish research activity, much of it in conjunction with Ross Anderson, then reader in epidemiology, and research was strengthened greatly by the recruitment of Bonnie Sibbald as research scientist. The first senior lecturer in general practice (Sean Hilton) was appointed in 1987, and a second in 1989 (Andre Tylee). In 1990 Fiona Ross was appointed senior lecturer in primary care nursing. Over the next three years the division of general practice grew steadily (Tony Kendrick, Pit Rink, Sally Kerry, Tess Harris, Pippa Oakeshott, Sangeeta Patel were added to the staff), and it was 'starred' in the 1991 RAE.

### Full department
Paul Freeling retired in 1993, and Sean Hilton was appointed professor and head of the now independent department of general practice and primary care. In the mid-1990s the department grew to its largest, with the infusion of funding that came as part of the 1994–1996 LIZEI programme. During that time membership rose from around thirty to between sixty and seventy, and Frank Smith was appointed as an additional senior lecturer to lead on a range of educational projects. Also in 1996, St George's combined with academic departments at King's and UMDS to set up StaRNet (South Thames Research Network).

### Assimilation back into Community Health Sciences Division
Gradually, however, an exodus of staff to chairs elsewhere began. Bonnie Sibbald moved to the National Primary Care Research and Development Centre in Manchester, where she made a distinguished contribution throughout its life. Departures accelerated after the 1996 RAE (Tony Kendrick, Fiona Ross, Andre Tylee and Frank Smith). A second chair in primary care research and development was awarded to

Franco Cappuccio in 1999. However, consequent on financial difficulties at the time, this was at the expense of the two clinical senior lecturer posts. The critical mass of general practitioners in the department was falling, and in 2002 the school restructuring of twenty-six separate departments into six large divisions led to the assimilation of general practice and primary care into the new division of community health sciences.

*Sean Hilton*

# UNIVERSITY COLLEGE LONDON MEDICAL SCHOOL

In 1998, the Royal Free Hospital Medical School merged with University College Hospital Medical School to become University College London Medical School.

## Royal Free Hospital

In 1877 the Royal Free Hospital became the first hospital in England to provide clinical training for women who had been students at the London School of Medicine for Women. The medical school was renamed the Royal Free Hospital School of Medicine in 1948. Thirty years later the hospital and medical school were finally united and re-located on a single site in Hampstead.

Establishing general practice as part of the undergraduate curriculum began in the late 1970s and early 1980s, although voluntary placements were offered to students in the 1950s by Philip Hopkins, a well-known Hampstead general practitioner. Twenty years later a teaching group was set up by Chris Donovan working with Mary Boothroyd Brooks, senior lecturer in public health. Chris, an Oxford PPE graduate and briefly a City merchant banker, had left his Hampstead general practice to work in the Edinburgh department, but soon returned to his old practice and became involved with the development of the Royal Free initiative. Sheila Sherlock was then professor of medicine and was not enamoured of local general practice, once asking Chris Donovan 'Why do you want to turn my students into social workers?'

Students in their second clinical year spent time in general practices in north London and had seminars in the medical school led by local general practitioners who were part-time senior lecturers. They were members of the department of clinical epidemiology and general practice headed by Gerry Shaper, a cardiovascular epidemiologist who set up the British Regional Heart Study. In 1983 he invited John Horder, recently president of the RCGP, to become visiting professor in general practice. John played a vital role in establishing general practice as an academic discipline in the medical school. With Shaper he successfully negotiated funding for a full-time lectureship in general practice which was established in 1986 and he continued to provide support and leadership for the eight years of his professorship.

The appointment of Margaret Lloyd as a full-time lecturer was the next step in building a group of academic general practitioners based on the original part-time senior lecturers. In 1990 Joe Rosenthal was appointed as a second full-time lecturer and teaching expanded. Students continued to have general practice attachments in their second and final clinical years, the latter provided by general practitioners around the country. The department introduced early patient contact for students in their first and second years and developed the teaching of communication skills which had been introduced by John Horder.

During the 1990s funding was sought for the establishment of a chair of general practice and David Cohen, a Hampstead general practitioner, agreed to fund a chair for seven years, after which it would be taken over by the medical school. In 1993 Paul Wallace was appointed the David Cohen professor of general practice, and the division of population and health care sciences was established which included the department of general practice and primary care. A decision not to have a general practice which was formally linked to the department had been made in the early years of its development and the lecturers and senior lecturers worked part-time in local practices.

In 1994 the Royal Free department of general practice merged with the department of primary care of University College London to become the department of primary care and population sciences, with Paul Wallace as its first head. This predated the merger of the two institutions in 1998 which had been proposed in the Tomlinson Report of 1993.

The joint department continued to be multidisciplinary and based on two sites, one at Archway close to the Whittington Hospital and the other in newly refurbished premises at the Royal Free. In 1998 Paul Wallace was succeeded as head of department by Andy Haines, followed by Michael Modell in 2000.

The teaching commitments of the two departments were complementary and developed further with the setting up in 1994 of the Community Based Medical Education in North Thames project involving all the medical schools in the North Thames Region. The project aimed to provide training and support for general practitioners to teach clinical

skills to undergraduates. General practitioners and hospital special-
ists worked together to design standards for teaching medicine in the
primary care setting. The project laid the foundation for the development
of community-based general medical teaching and the establishment
of a group of university-linked practices. These practices had a regular
commitment to taking students with the general practitioners having
protected time for teaching. Further developments included the introduction in 1997 of an intercalated BSc in primary health care for medical
students and the expansion of courses for practice nurses. These courses
had been set up by Mary Walker, a senior research nurse involved with
the British Regional Heart Study and a number of academic appointments in nursing were later established within the department.

The primary care research activities of the Royal Free department
developed after the appointment of Paul Wallace and initially focused
on the application of telemedicine to the primary care interface with
secondary care. The merger of the two departments led to further expansion of multidisciplinary research activities in primary care including
the study of factors influencing behaviour change, community genetics,
the impact of environmental factors on health and the setting up of the
North Central Thames Primary Care Research Network.

*Margaret Lloyd*
*Chris Donovan*

## University College Hospital

In the mid-1960s University College Hospital Medical School (UCHMS)
was a traditional teaching hospital-based London medical school with
an annual entry of about 100, mainly white middle-class males. Students
spent the first two years of the course studying the basic sciences, with
next to no patient contact. Three years of clinical training followed,
centred on UCH, with a few months spent at other hospitals and no
obligatory community attachments (apart from a day visiting a general
practice and the public baths). A few senior students chose to spend a
week or two attached to a local practice.

There was no concept of academic primary care as was inevitable at
a time when most doctors who entered general practice had little postgraduate training and there was an almost complete absence of high
quality general practitioner-based research. The vast majority of senior
medical staff had minimal experience of general practice, and general
practitioners were often perceived as doctors who could not make the
grade in hospital medicine. This view was sustained by the poor quality

of some inner-city medical practice. From 1966 to 1969 all paediatric students spent half a day with me visiting children with rashes; this was their sole official general practice attachment. This began after one paediatric house officer had admitted a child with early measles, causing consternation on the ward. She then complained that she had never seen children in the prodromal stage of that disease – a very common illness in the days before routine immunisation. Obligatory second clinical year general practice attachments began in 1969, with one week in a practice outside London and the other attached either to the Caversham or the James Wigg group practices (both destined to join the Kentish Town Health Centre in 1973). The medical school had already developed a close relationship with these practices, although they never became university practices.

I was appointed as the tutor in general practice at the end of 1971, with an honorarium of £500 per annum. I was responsible for arranging the students' general practice attachments, and seen as the main link between the school and the other local practices. Within a few years the general practice unit (GPU) was formed and other general practitioners were appointed as recognised teachers. Another achievement of those early years, under the guidance of John Horder, was the establishment at UCH of one of the first London three-year general practice vocational training schemes – naturally linked to the Kentish Town Health Centre. The rest of the decade was a struggle, first to gain recognition and respect, second to increase the resources available to teaching practices, and third to increase the amount of time students spent with general practitioners. The early general practice tutors knew that they had to establish their credibility and were prepared to spend a considerable amount of time with students for next to no payment. Here I must pay tribute to that little band of early UCL enthusiasts including the partners in Kentish Town Health Centre and Tony Antoniou, Simon Wiseman, Melvin Ross and Robert MacGibbon. The philosophy of the GPU was that, in the context of undergraduate teaching, general practice should be viewed both as the practice of medicine in the community and as a specific discipline on a par with the other clinical subjects. Appropriately, the unit became part of the department of medicine rather than joining a department of public health and epidemiology, which was seen by some tutors as a non-clinical subject.

The attitude of the medical school staff to academic primary care was ambivalent. Some, including the Dean, Arthur Prophet, were supportive, but others were less enthusiastic. This was exemplified by a letter received in 1979 from a senior professor following yet another rather desperate request from me for more money. It included phrases such as 'trying to put a pistol to the head of the medical school' and a description of my request as 'reminiscent of "my last territorial demand"'. Nevertheless, by the end of the decade our funding had risen to about £16,000 per annum. By then clinical students spent a month attached to general practices with a minor input into other parts of the curriculum. The unit consisted of two part-time senior lecturers, three part-time lecturers, a secretary and a gradually increasing number of Camden and Islington teaching practices.

By 1980 UCHMS had become the School of Medicine UCL and the College was now keen to take advantage of any funded opportunity that might arise to expand academic primary care. The main tasks of the early 1980s were to join with the Middlesex Hospital GPU, headed since 1981 by John Cohen, to start a research programme, and to move towards a department of primary care led by a general practitioner with a respected research track record. The two units became a 'virtual' joint sub-department a couple of years before the two medical schools officially merged in the mid-1980s. This pattern of early very close collaboration between neighbouring sub-departments of primary care was repeated ten years later in the two years before the Royal Free Hospital School of Medicine joined UCL. We were fully aware at the beginning of that decade of two possible academic weaknesses of the GPU. First it was focused almost entirely on general practice rather than the wider concept of primary care; second it was staffed solely by busy 'jobbing' general practitioners none of whom had received a traditional academic training in research methodology. This meant that research had to come a poor second to teaching and we still had a problem of credibility within UCL, though not (according to opinion surveys) with medical students. However, we did obtain extra funding mainly from the NHS and the university to appoint two researchers, Jenny Harding and Mary Bollam.

The earliest research projects leading to papers in peer-reviewed journals were all centred on the local north London general practices and focused on patient care rather than epidemiology. The subjects covered included patients' assessment of out of hours care, the evaluation of a management plan for patients with asthma, elderly peoples' perception of discharge from hospital, and the use of an Alcometer to detect problem drinkers. In February 1984, UCL was awarded a grant of £45,000 per annum from the University Academic Initiatives Scheme towards the establishment of a department of primary health care. Inevitably, it was envisaged that part of the funding would come from the NHS and several members of the staff would be general practitioners with part-time academic appointments. Then followed two years of sometimes painful negotiations in the working party on primary health care around the job description for the new professor. The staff of the GPU felt strongly that the new head should have a background in clinical primary care, whereas the College doubted whether there were sufficient applicants with the necessary academic track record. Perhaps the post could be filled by someone from another medical discipline? One member of the working party wondered whether an epidemiologist from Uppsala was a possibility. Our 1985–1986 Jephcott professor, David Metcalfe from Manchester, became embroiled in this struggle, as did some of our local eminent general practitioners. Fortunately, in October 1986 Andy Haines – a general practitioner with research interests in epidemiology and primary care HSR and then at St Mary's – was appointed to the chair.

The space provided in the medical school reflected the status of the subject. Until the mid-1970s the 'department' was a desk in a school secretary's office. Then followed ten years in a small office in an outpost on the central site, sharing a teaching room with the even smaller sub-department of community medicine. Finally, we spent another decade in various temporary buildings, until we ended up in a renovated ward at the Archway campus. In spite of that, the progress between 1986 and 1994 was very considerable, the department blossoming both in research and teaching. With the arrival of Andy the department developed in a more academically traditional way, the focus shifting from the local teaching practices to the university site. His priority was to build up research expertise and this led in the early years to the appointment of Irwin Nazareth, Elizabeth Murray and Trish Greenhalgh and a substantial programme of health service research including care of the elderly (Iliffe, Haines and others), telemedicine (Wallace, Haines and others), shared decision-making (Murray, Haines and others), evaluation of a pharmacy care plan for elderly patients being discharged from hospital (Nazareth and Haines and others) and a range of projects on mental health in primary care led by Irwin Nazareth.

By 1990 several hospitals within Bloomsbury had been closed, in-patient stays were getting shorter and the school became receptive to the proposal that junior clinical students could be taught basic clinical skills by general practitioners. The Dean, Professor John Pattison, was sympathetic, and provided funding (before SIFT came on-stream for general practice) to establish in 1994 a five-week first clinical year 'medicine in the community' firm replacing one based in the hospital. Between 1993 and 1996 Andy Haines was seconded as Director of R&D to the North Thames Region and this raised the profile of primary care within the NHS R&D programme generally.

The department merged with the Royal Free Hospital School of Medicine department led by Paul Wallace, who in 1996 became the first head of the merged department of primary care and population sciences. He was followed by Andy Haines until the latter became director of the London School of Hygiene and Tropical Medicine in 2000.

Links with primary care departments overseas were developed, most notably in Brazil, where visits to Porto Alegre in particular and to the ministry of health in Brasilia proved influential at a time when the Brazilians were beginning to develop their own family health programme in the late 1980s and early 1990s. This has now expanded to cover over 100 million people. The international course run by the department has trained a number of international leaders in primary care.

*Michael Modell*
*Andy Haines*

# Chapter 21

# The University of St Andrews

In any research project, there is always one subject that seems to defy classification! On this occasion it is the University of St Andrews. Although it has taught medical students for nearly 600 years and thus cannot be regarded as a 'new' medical school (as covered in Appendix 1 which follows this chapter), it did not have a department of general practice during the lifetime of the AUTGP.

In many ways it is particularly fitting that St Andrews should be included here as the last chapter in the main body of our Histories, as it is where Sir James Mackenzie, general practitioner and cardiologist and rightly regarded as the first true academic general practitioner, retired to in 1919 to establish his Institute of Clinical Research, arguably the first ever department of general practice anywhere. And it was from his and his daughter Dorothy's estates that the first chair of general practice in Edinburgh was endowed.

*The editors*

## University of St Andrews

Although a 'new department', St Andrews, through James Mackenzie, can almost certainly lay claim to having had one of the first, if not the first, departments of academic general practice. In 1919, Sir James, who believed that general practice was the proper place for clinical research, managed to enlist the support and help of every general practitioner in the town in collaborating in clinical research. Following Mackenzie's death his Institute suffered funding difficulties and eventually closed its doors in 1944.

The rebirth of academic general practice at St Andrews occurred in 2008 with the appointment of Cathy Jackson to its first chair in primary care medicine. The need for the department arose from the new requirement of St Andrews medical students to move after three years to one of five clinical partner schools, rather than just to Manchester as previously, and for the university to ensure that students had had the appropriate clinical experience to join any one of them. It was also necessary to meet the learning outcomes required by the GMC document *Tomorrow's Doctors*.

By 2010 over forty general practitioners in Fife and Tayside had become involved in the St Andrews' clinical teaching programme, with further expansion to other areas of Scotland planned for 2011. Also by 2010 development of infrastructure for primary care research at St Andrews was well underway, not only using networks of established academics but also successfully encouraging 'coal face' general practitioners to put forward and develop ideas in a bid to make a research and teaching culture the norm for practices in Fife.

*Cathy Jackson*

# Appendix 1 Primary Care in the New Medical Schools

Medical student numbers have grown steadily during the life of the NHS. Apart from the creation of the new schools of the 1960s (Leicester, Nottingham and Southampton), the increase in places has been achieved by opportunistic distribution throughout the long-established medical schools. However, between 1998 and 2005, the government created seven further medical schools to accommodate its most recent plans to increase student numbers. The notes that follow describe how this has been achieved.

*John Campbell*

## Brighton and Sussex Medical School

Brighton and Sussex Medical School (BSMS) has two parent universities, the University of Sussex (part of the first wave of 1960s universities) and the University of Brighton (founded in the 1990s with a strong professional focus).

General practice lives within the division of primary care and public health, one of three departments within the medical school, the others being clinical medicine and clinical and laboratory investigation. BSMS trades on its smallness (680 students), its integrated course, strong student support and innovative anatomy teaching (that does include dissection). After three cohorts of graduates, it has progressed from being a 'new' to a 'young' school, and delights in being amongst the top three most popular medical schools with students.

Helen Smith was appointed to the foundation chair of primary care in 2003, six months ahead of the first cohort of students arriving. The task of curriculum development in such a tight window was facilitated by the purchase of the Southampton curriculum. This was significantly modified to reflect BSMS's own ideology and to incorporate best current practice. Although 'general practice' does not appear formally in the BSMS curriculum until years four and five, it makes a broad contribution to teaching, throughout the entire five years. This is facilitated by there being no divide between non-clinical and clinical phases, and also by the inability of secondary care to provide sufficient suitable patients for teaching. Working with students on their portfolios and early clinical case reports and acting as personal tutors, general practitioners play an important role in the students' professional development. General practice also contributes to the teaching of student-selected components and the supervision of individual research projects.

In year four, students have their first formal general practice attachment – a long, thin module with half-day seminars and general practice placements scattered between attachment to the '-ologies'. In year five the attachment is more traditional, with a four-week block in a regional centre.

Research studies blend epidemiology, clinical and health services research with a multidisciplinary research group with expertise in general practice, health psychology, statistics, anthropology, nutrition, public health, epidemiology, computing and information technology. The division also hosts the NIHR primary care research network for the south-east. In the early life of the division it was essential to be responsive to the research needs of the wider health community and a rather eclectic research portfolio developed. However, with other research groups established in other specialities able to share this research support role, research strategy is more focused. For the next five years the programme of work will address under-researched areas in sexual health, cancer, allergy and the general practice electronic patient record.

*Helen Smith*

## Hull York Medical School

This new medical school was established in 2002 as a joint venture between the universities of Hull and York. Two chairs in primary care in Hull and York predated the formation of the new school and were established in the 1990s. Peter Campion was appointed in Hull alongside developments which saw the university extend its interest in health and health care with the establishment of the Hull postgraduate medical institute. Ian Watt was the first professor of primary care in the University of York which became part of a new multidisciplinary department of health sciences.

Hull York Medical School (HYMS) developed a new and innovative curriculum with half of the course delivered in primary care, problem-based learning and early clinical contact. This is a spiral curriculum based on seven themes (including patient-centred care and population health) running throughout the five years of the course.

HYMS has no discipline-based departments. Instead most academic staff, whilst undertaking teaching responsibilities in HYMS, are placed in pre-existing departments in both universities for their research activities. In York, Ian Watt, as professor of primary care, researches with colleagues in the department of health sciences. Approximately half of the research undertaken in the department of health sciences is focused on primary care, and in the last RAE the department was ranked joint first in the UK for HSR.

General practitioners are well represented within the medical school in a range of positions. The Dean (Professor Tony Kendrick), and the undergraduate school Dean (Professor David Blaney) are both general practitioners. In Hull, Peter Campion retired in 2010 and was replaced by Una Macleod.

*Peter Campion*


## Peninsula Medical School

Peninsula Medical School was established in 2002, incorporating the postgraduate medical schools in Exeter and Plymouth. Denis Pereira Gray had established Exeter as a leading international centre of post-graduate general practice training. More recently, Frank Dobbs had been appointed as clinical senior lecturer in primary care in Plymouth, leading primary care research in that locality. Professor John Tooke, the first Dean of the Peninsula undergraduate medical school, brought together the academic and NHS resources in the south-west within the new school, which has been extended by securing a dental school now integrated within the Peninsula College of Medicine and Dentistry.

In 2002, John Campbell was appointed as foundation chair in general practice and primary care, moving from King's College London. In 2010, a second chair in primary care diagnostics was created, with Professor Willie Hamilton moving from the University of Bristol. The current refurbished premises in the Smeall Building on the St Luke's Campus of the University of Exeter have potential for significant future growth.

The model for undergraduate medical education adopted in the Peninsula separated research from undergraduate education. Management responsibilities for the primary care undergraduate programme rest with the community sub-Deans, Steve Watkins, Colan

Robinson and Alex Harding, and around 20 per cent of the undergraduate programme is delivered in community settings. The undergraduate programme itself is strongly problem-based with a spirally integrated curriculum. There are no distinct academic departments. From an initial cohort of around eighty students per year, Peninsula now has an annual intake of 215 students with thirteen overseas students forming part of the annual cohort. Admissions criteria are directly competitive with other UK leading medical schools, and the 2009 National Student Survey ranked Peninsula in joint first position for student experience (along with Oxford, Edinburgh and Brighton and Sussex). The undergraduate programme involves four assessment modules – applied medical knowledge, clinical skills, professionalism and student-selected components. The use of progress testing of applied medical knowledge is highly innovative, replicating models which have only been previously exploited in Maastricht and McMaster. In this model, all students from all years for the undergraduate programme undertake the same knowledge assessment on four occasions each year. Inevitably, junior students, having previously been used to scoring highly in other academic settings, find themselves with very low scores in the early years of the undergraduate programme. However, the intent is to demonstrate growth in knowledge and this is clearly demonstrated for the vast majority of students over a five-year period. The assessment programme was introduced by John Bligh, formerly Vice-Dean (education).

Research within the medical school, the principal provenance of John Campbell and his team, has grown substantially since 2002. The principal focus is on accessibility and quality of primary care provision. Other major themes include the evaluation and assessment of patients at risk of cardiovascular disease, including those with early diabetes diagnosed in primary care settings. Finally, there is a developing interest in the management of patients with mental health problems in primary care settings. Much of the primary care research undertaken is collaborative, including associations with the universities of Plymouth, Exeter, Bristol, Cambridge and the RAND Corporation in the USA. In addition, a programme supporting seven academic clinical fellows is funded through the 'Walport' programme.

*John Campbell*

## University of East Anglia School of Medicine

Based in Norwich, the East Anglia School was formed in 2001 with the first students arriving in 2002. There are 170 students in each year with a high proportion of graduates. Amanda Howe is the inaugural professor of primary care. Practices and lead tutors are selected for their ability to provide an effective educational experience, and general practice teaching has been the most consistently highly evaluated component of the programme from the start.

Like the other new medical schools, the course normally lasts the standard five years and is an integrated course with no pre-clinical–clinical divide. It is a case-based course with consistent integration of theoretical learning and clinical practice. The main educational method is problem-based learning in peer groups of ten, underpinned by self-directed learning, with lectures and seminars as a resource. Students undertake all clinical placements in primary and secondary care, and also clinical and consultation skills training in the same peer group, with a consistent membership for one year.

Many varieties of assessment are used, including student selected topics which require 'conference style' activities: short oral presentations, abstracts, posters, grand round, and research projects. There is a reflective essay, inter-professional learning projects, and summative tutor reports from primary care and the problem-based learning group tutors. Other more conventional assessments are short notes, essays and Objective Structured Clinical Examinations.

*Amanda Howe*

## University of Keele

Keele University was founded in 1949, and although the undergraduate medical school is a new arrival, academic general practice at Keele has a longer history. In 1979, the nearby Stoke-on-Trent conurbation created a lively university postgraduate department of medicine. Wolstanton Medical Centre in Newcastle-under-Lyme was home to Alistair Ross (the first senior lecturer in general practice at Keele), Mike Fisher (whose vision created a novel academic framework for general practice vocational training based on Masters modules delivered at Keele), Peter Croft (who started the research-based primary care sciences centre), and Mark Shapley (now senior research fellow).

Brian McGuiness came to Keele in 1988 as reader in general practice and was awarded a personal chair four years later. He started a Masters in medical science to introduce trainee specialist doctors to aspects of general practice. It became the vehicle for the delivery of the academic vocational training programme, led by Mike Fisher and by Vince Cooper, senior lecturer in general practice. By 2005 this programme provided the basis for Keele's successful application for the NIHR academic fellows and clinical lectureships in general practice, and nurtured two of our current senior lecturers (Christian Mallen and Umesh Kadam).

During the 1990s, NHS investment from the North Staffordshire District Health Authority and local fund-holding general practices supported Peter Croft, Elaine Hay (the first academic community rheumatologist in England) and Rhian Hughes (a senior manager) in building the general practice research networks and the partnerships with hospital and community health services which formed the basis for Keele's research programme in pain and musculoskeletal disease.

### From 2000

In 2001, Keele was awarded an undergraduate medical school in partnership with Manchester University. The appointment of the first senior lecturer in general practice (Andy Bartlam) was followed by Bob McKinley's move from Leicester to the foundation chair of general practice in 2007. He joined Richard Hays from Australia, who had become the second head of the medical school, and Kay Mohanna, a general practitioner and director of postgraduate studies. When Richard returned to Australia in 2009, another general practitioner, Val Wass, was appointed head of school.

Keele is on the brink of becoming a fully independent school, the last students studying the Manchester curriculum at Keele graduating in 2011. The role of general practice at Keele is broadening as the number of clinical placements increase, including fifteen weeks in the final year. The school currently employs more general practitioners than any other clinical speciality, including six general practice senior lecturers, and shares its flagship building on the Keele campus with primary care sciences, which is now the largest research group in the faculty of health. This growth reflects thirty years of association with SAPC, from when Alistair Ross, one of that inspirational cohort of Scottish graduate general practitioners, was the lone Keele representative in AUDGP.

*Robert McKinley*

### University of Swansea

Swansea medical school offers a four-year graduate entry programme in medicine, with a current yearly intake of seventy-two students. Opening its doors to its first cohort in 2004, with a two-year programme shared with Cardiff medical school, Swansea now provides a full four-year programme in medical education. Community-based learning is an innovative and integrated aspect of this new programme currently compromising about 10 per cent of the taught curriculum.

The school aims to ensure educational integration between school-based teaching and community-based (general practice) experiential learning, whereby the teaching and learning in the community reinforces and anchors the topics of the case-based learning delivered by the school. A major aim of the community-based learning component of the programme is to inspire the students to recognise at an early stage of their career the benefits of self-directive learning and life-long professional development. This strand notably offers generic training and is not specific to primary care but highly relevant to core student training as defined by the GMC.

Currently students attend a named primary care centre for ten full days in their first and second years and for thirteen days in their third year. At the end of their final year, it is planned that students will be attached to a general practice for five weeks, immediately before they commence work on the wards as new doctors. Training of the community-based learning tutors from amongst the primary care physicians and monitoring of student experience and training in the community is ongoing and rigorous, ensuring a highly enjoyable student experience and adding a successful component to this new and innovative graduate entry programme.

*Mary Hoptroff*

## University of Warwick

In the early 1990s, two part-time honorary clinical senior lecturers (John Wilmot and Roger Gadsby) were appointed to the school of postgraduate medical education, funded by the West Midlands deanery. John Wilmot became course director of the MSc in primary care management, and Roger Gadsby became course director of the certificate in diabetes care.

Jeremy Dale was appointed as foundation professor of primary care in 1997 to establish and lead a centre for primary care research and teaching. His post was funded by the Coventry and Warwickshire Health Authorities. In 1998, with further funding from the West Midlands deanery, the centre for primary health care studies was launched, with Frances Griffiths appointed as a clinical senior lecturer and Hilary Hearnshaw as senior lecturer.

The centre for primary health care studies was a free-standing research centre, and as such managed its own budget. It rapidly developed new income-generating courses, particularly related to diabetes. In 2000 it launched Warwick Diabetes Care. It also launched several MSc courses and a diploma in occupational health. These funded growth in the administrative and teaching teams, and enabled the appointment of primary care academics, including Rodger Charlton. Growth in the centre's research programme was supported by infrastructure funding from West Midlands NHS R&D, and in 2000 Warwick and Coventry Primary Care Research was established.

In 2000, Warwick medical school was launched, initially as part of Leicester Warwick medical school. Rodger Charlton became the lead for undergraduate general practice teaching at Warwick, and was soon joined by Teresa Pawlikowska.

Jeremy Dale played a key role in the early development of the school, acting as Vice-Dean prior to the appointment of Yvonne Carter. He was instrumental in promoting the early academic appointments, including the chairs of public health (Sarah Stewart Brown), epidemiology (Margaret Thorogood), mental health (Scott Weich), so ensuring that the school had a particularly strong primary care orientation in its early years. While still remaining as a distinct entity, the centre for primary health care studies (CPHCS) became the core element of the division of health in the community, with Jeremy Dale as its head.

In 2004, Yvonne Carter became Vice-Dean and began to apply her tremendous energy and vision to the development of the medical school. As the school quickly grew, re-structuring became inevitable, with teaching and research being split into separate divisions. Eventually in 2007, CPHCS was disbanded as new structures took forward its research activities, its teaching courses having become part of the Institute of Clinical Education some years earlier.

*Jeremy Dale*

## Further reading

Howe A., Campion P., Searle J. and Smith H., 'New perspectives – approaches to medical education at four new UK medical schools', *BMJ*, 328, 2004: 327–32.

# Appendix 2  The SIFT/ACT Negotiations

The aims and constitution of the original AUTGP were drafted to promote the academic development of the discipline. The intention was that there should not be any significant element of 'trade union' activity, but the problems consequent on the totally insufficient funding of the early departments by their universities and medical schools surfaced regularly at the early executive committee meetings.

Across the NHS generally, the Department of Health was attempting to find a more explicit and more equitable formula for distributing its resources. This led in 1974 to the publication of the Resource Allocation Working Party (RAWP) Report, identifying historical differences between the total costs of running 'teaching' and 'non-teaching' hospitals. These differences were rationalised as being due to the 'service costs of teaching' (SIFT) and put back into the subsequent funding formula on a 'per clinical student per year' basis. From the outset these funds were payable only to hospitals. General-practice-based teaching was excluded, and so began our campaign for the provision of an analogous subsidy to meet the extra costs of supporting academic costs in the clinical setting of general practice. In 1974 the sum identified as needed to support hospital-based academic work was around £8,000 per student per year – a sum which had grown to nearly £40,000 per year (nearly £5 billion for the NHS nationally) by the time that first teaching practices (1990) and then departments of general practice (1992) won a share of NHS support funding.

In December 1981, the heads of departments of general practice in England and Scotland wrote to the CMOs of their respective Departments of Health asking for a share of SIFT or of ACT (the 'addition for clinical teaching', the Scottish equivalent of SIFT) to underpin academic costs and activity in general practice, or for access to equivalent support. It was to be ten years later (December 1991) before the key meeting within the DH which confirmed success in our quest. (In fact we still await definitive answers to our letters of 1981!)

The negotiation that followed was to have three parts to it: making a case, finding a mechanism to implement it, and identifying a resource to fund that implementation. Although the three parts went roughly in that order, we often found ourselves having to restart at the beginning when new officials took over, or when the discussions were moved from one part of government to another. The early events in the campaign centred round attempts by the Departments of Health and of Education to shift responsibility for lack of progress from one to the other – a process that at one time seemed destined to be played out for ever. The Health Departments found a further problem; their lawyers believed it would be illegal to use NHS money to support teaching in general practice as the 1978 NHS Act had limited the Secretary of State's responsibility for supporting teaching to costs incurred in hospitals. In 1983, a carefully planned meeting at the King's Fund in London brought key players from the academic and NHS communities together for the first time and helpfully outlined the nature and size of the problem ahead. However, after two further years of rather aimless shadow boxing, the need for a formal document to support our negotiations became apparent and this led in 1986 to the publication of the Mackenzie Report.[1] Following its wide circulation, various initiatives gathered the essential momentum we had never until then adequately succeeded in creating.

Early in 1987, Michael Colvin, a (Conservative) government backbench MP, was introduced to the fray by George Freeman and he provided a significant boost to our campaign with a parliamentary question to the DH within an hour of his agreeing to help. The pace quickened. Alastair Riddell, then chairman of Scottish GMSC and one of the profession's negotiators, offered what proved to be critically important guidance and support. He warned of the need not to miss an expected decennial NHS 'primary legislation' opportunity, and this led to an upsurge in political activity. Increasingly hectic discussions led to an adjournment debate in Parliament (October 1987), and from there to an enabling clause in the 1989 Health and Medicines Bill through which GMS payments for teaching ('paragraph 40') became a reality in the 'New GP Contract' of 1990.

However, the all-important 'infrastructure' support for departments of general practice, which had throughout been an equal thrust in our negotiations, remained as a 'pending' item. Through David Metcalfe's membership of the 'France Committee' (the Standing Group on Medical and Dental Education and Research – SGUMDER), and later through the work of its parallel Working Group (WGUMDER), we continued to press our case throughout the early 1990s. When SGUMDER agreed to set up a dedicated working party to 'explore mechanisms' for addressing the problem of how to support academic general practice we had victory in sight, as the question of 'the case' had apparently been accepted and was no longer to be an issue. An unexpectedly good PES (Public Expenditure Settlement) in 1991 led to Department of Health officials suggesting that we used a mechanism called 'tasking' of RHAs, which was available at that time and required regions to carry out central policy wishes from within their own budgets. Through this mechanism the first 'tasked money' was identified and became available. In due course, 'GP SIFT/ACT' became a formula-driven sum and went on to provide exactly what we had set out to achieve more than a decade earlier.

What lessons can we learn from this story? First, that the Treasury holds the key to everything with financial implications. Second, that the Treasury can only be approached through Under-Secretaries. And third, that Under-Secretaries are moved every three years or so, so the process is difficult to enter or to influence. 'Yes, Minister' is accurate and is essential watching! Success is ultimately about who supports you and who has influence; about who is blocking you or has a conflicting agenda; and about whether those who appear to give support in public are in fact those who block in private. It is about understanding the processes of government, about sensing windows of opportunity; and about playing a long game and accepting reverses with equanimity. Above all, the story is about persistence – and about having strong beliefs, and strong support from others sharing the same goals and contributing information and ideas to the campaign.

It is difficult to write an article like this without referring to many who have played key roles. John Horder, before and after his time as president of the RCGP, was a strong and important emissary throughout. Three English and three Scottish CMOs and several PMOs played important roles, and of them Donald Acheson and Geoffrey Rivett were more involved than others. Four Under-Secretaries, and some more junior and several more senior civil servants played central parts. David Morrell at the start of RAWP, John Walker and David Metcalfe between 1980 and 1990, and George Freeman and John Bain – whose contacts with Michael Colvin (our backbench MP) were so important – along with Alastair Riddell and successive GMSC negotiators put essential parts of the jigsaw together. But in the end, it was the case itself that won the day!

*John Howie*
(Adapted from the SAPC Newsletter, August 2005)

## Note

1. Howie J.G.R., Hannay D.R. and Stevenson J.S.K., *The Mackenzie Report: General Practice in the Medical Schools of the United Kingdom – 1986*, Edinburgh, University of Edinburgh, 1986.

## Further reading

Howie J.G.R., *Patient-centredness and the Politics of Change*, The Nuffield Trust, London, 1999, Chapter 3, pp. 25–76.

# *Appendix 3  An Overview*

The year 2008 marked the sixtieth anniversary of the founding of the NHS. The first academic department of general practice in the modern era also dated from the 'due date' for the start of the NHS on 1 July, when the University of Edinburgh established its 'academic general practice' in the former Mackenzie House Public Dispensary within its department of social medicine. By 2000, there were twenty-nine departments of general practice in the traditional medical schools of the UK (the department in Trinity College Dublin has traditionally been included in this grouping). The history of their evolution and development has been interesting but not always straightforward; often a source of frustration but eventually one of achievement and satisfaction. This essay tries to tease out some of the issues that have had to be faced up to on the journey.

## Timelines

### *Within the UK*

Following the birth of the NHS in 1948, the highly critical Collings Report of 1950[1] led to the foundation in 1952 of the College of General Practitioners, one of whose first aims was to see established a department of general practice in every UK medical school. The Edinburgh department became independent in 1956 and its chair followed in 1963. Between 1970 and 1972 three other chairs were established in Scotland. Manchester (1972) led the way in England, but it took until 1995 for all schools to follow. From 1971 onwards regional (postgraduate) advisers were appointed in all UK regions, mostly with connections to medical schools through postgraduate Deans. In Exeter, a postgraduate chair was established in 1986.

The emerging cohort of undergraduate departments held its first scientific meeting in 1972 in Cardiff, and the AUTGP was established as its scientific society in 1974 (later becoming the AUDGP and – in 2000 – SAPC). Although these organisations were constituted as scientific organisations, their members (originally – but no longer – mainly doctors) also saw their existence as necessary to take forward structural agendas that were not being sufficiently addressed elsewhere. Of greatest importance was the absence of adequate and equitable core funding from either the NHS or the university funding systems, in marked contrast to the very considerable NHS budgets available to support postgraduate education and the regional adviser infrastructure. The negotiations to address this problem took from 1981 until 1992, and their successful conclusion with the establishment of 'GP SIFT' in England and the parallel 'GP ACT' in Scotland marked a watershed in the capacity of undergraduate departments to flourish and achieve their potential. During these protracted negotiations, the GMSC of the BMA was particularly helpful in opening negotiating channels to the then DHSS.

### Abroad

It is easy to view the evolution of academic general practice from a narrow UK perspective. However, the world's second chair was established in 1966 in Utrecht, and its holder (Jan van Es) referred to the mushrooming of chairs around the north Atlantic countries as a process of 'simultaneity'.[2] Ian McWhinney was appointed to his chair at the University of Western Ontario in 1967. Europe developed its own academic institution SIMG in 1962, and WONCA was inaugurated in 1972. In 1974, the Leeuwenhorst Group (defining the discipline of general practice) and the EGPRW were created. The European bodies amalgamated as WONCA Europe in 1996.

### Organisations and structures

Several structural events have greatly influenced the evolution of general practice in the UK. The 1966 'Charter' opened the way for the construction of modern general practice by encouraging the development of group practices and the employment of interdisciplinary and clerical staffing. 1990 saw the twin initiatives of general practice fund-holding and the institution (imposition) of a then 'New Contract'. This was replaced in 2004 by the present Contract. Patients are now registered with practices rather than a personal doctor; doctors have largely opted out of twenty-four-hour responsibility for patient care; and the QOF payment structure has shifted the emphasis at consultations away from giving priority to the agendas of patients towards meeting targets which, inter alia, relate to the generation of practice income.

In 1973, the MRC established its GPRN to help recruit patients for national studies it was supporting. The JCPTGP was created in 1975 – the AUDGP having one representative on it – and vocational training for general practice became mandatory in 1982. The DH established the NPCRDC in Manchester in 1996.

These overlapping sets of dates show how many and how complex have been the influences surrounding academic general practice and its evolution over sixty years.

## A university discipline and its purpose

There have been several attempts to define the criteria of a university clinical discipline. Two are closely similar, by McWhinney in 1966[3] and by Richardson in 1975.[4] Both included the presence of a unique body of knowledge, having specific clinical skills, and the ability to support original research in their sets of four key criteria. McWhinney's fourth criterion was the ability of the discipline to manage its own postgraduate training; Richardson's was the possession of a philosophy. From a different perspective, Pereira Gray has argued that a subject becomes an academic discipline when it has its own literature.[5]

Those who work in clinical disciplines also provide service care, and many of the early departments were constructed round busy inner-city practices with a heavy workload. In 1986, the Mackenzie Report described the juxtaposition of medical schools and service general practice in this way: 'Universities are hierarchical organisations whereas general practice is strongly egalitarian; Universities emphasise research and theory, whereas general practice has evolved from experience and instinct.'[6] One important role of 'academic general practice' (defined for the present purpose as the undergraduate departments in the traditional medical schools) has been to build bridges between the two very different cultures of medical schools and service general practice. Four areas of work have been involved: teaching about medicine in the setting of the community; carrying out research to establish the nature of general practice and to improve delivery of clinical care; contributing to the organisation and administration of universities and the NHS; and contributing to the wider philosophy of medical practice and its role in society. Have the departments of general practice succeeded in these roles?

Within medical schools, the answer must be 'yes'. Around 15 per cent of the undergraduate curriculum is now taught under the supervision of departments of general practice. General practice research figured prominently in the RAEs of 1992, 1996 and 2001, although – significantly – its identity was compromised in the 2008 RAE when the research output from around half of all general practice researchers was declared within research categories other than general practice. The undergraduate departments have contributed strongly to the literature of the discipline and thus to the creation of the current evidence base of clinical practice. Their staff have been prominent in the wider life of medical school administration, and there and elsewhere have contributed significantly to the evolving understanding of the relationships between medicine and society.

## Three tensions

The histories of the developing departments tell of individuals with vision, drive and perseverance who overcame many obstacles on the way to achieving their aims. They say relatively little about those with power or influence who were either positively obstructive or simply failed to show the leadership that could have made progress so much easier.

Three more general issues added to the difficulties faced by the emerging discipline.

### 'Real doctors' or 'real academics'?

Certainly in the early years, but probably less so now, there has been a tension over whether academic general practitioners were proper doctors or proper academics. Many early academic staff would have claimed public health as their basic clinical discipline, and service general practitioners were unconvinced of their ability to speak the language of 'ordinary' doctors. Even those coming to universities from a clearly general practice background lost credibility when their responsibilities for patients became diminished, particularly through their inability to provide either continuing or comprehensive care. At the same time, the appointment of doctors to senior university posts without higher research degrees or significant records of contribution to peer-reviewed literature created scepticism within universities, compounded by the award to them of top clinical salaries against the prevailing lower incomes of academic staff in other faculties and of non-clinical staff in medical faculties.

Most of the first departments were built around service general practices staffed mainly or exclusively by university-employed staff (who were paid on the non-consultant clinical scales). The hope (of universities) was that income generated from patient care would contribute significantly to the costs of these departments, but service income never proved able to support an adequate academic infrastructure. In addition, although list sizes were normally smaller than standard, the very nature of the direct availability of doctors in general practice to their patients resulted in clinical work taking priority over academic work, often confirming the view of those in other academic disciplines that academic general practice lacked academic credibility. On the other hand, a number of departments (now virtually all) were created on the assumption that academic staff would develop separate clinical connections with existing local practices. This has created a different set of contractual difficulties (there is still no equivalent of an honorary consultant in a hospital discipline) for academic general practitioners. The clinical credibility of those holding such posts has depended on their personal track records as family doctors, but their academic output has tended to be more substantial than was that of many of those in the early 'practice-based' departments.

### Undergraduate and postgraduate medicine

At the local level, undergraduate and postgraduate general practice has normally (but not always) integrated well. Many early vocational training programmes were created from within undergraduate departments, and day-release programmes have gained much from the contributions of those actively involved in research in the undergraduate setting. In many places, research training posts were created under the auspices of postgraduate medicine and funding, but housed and supervised within the undergraduate departments. Undergraduate staff have also contributed significantly to the continuing education of general practitioners.

At the national and political level, the need for undergraduate and postgraduate departments to establish their own spheres of influence has sometimes created tensions. The establishment of the AUTGP was a response to the emergence of needs and priorities within the university system which were different from those of the RCGP. The relative distancing of regional advisers from undergraduate departments reflected the reality that supervision of vocational training had become a major role for the RCGP and for many of its leading figures, replacing the College's role in its early years as a driver of undergraduate education attachments and of general practice research. Nonetheless, at a personnel level, many leading players have had multiple roles, exemplified by the writing of *The Future General Practitioner* in 1972,[7] published by the BMA, but the result of an RCGP working party, most of whose members were or became leading 'academic' thinkers. The development of the membership examination for the RCGP was another good example of joint working between members of the undergraduate and postgraduate communities.

One consequence of the different paths followed by the College and the university departments has been their very different involvements in international academic affairs. While the College took a significant role in the development SIMG, the Leeuwenhorst Group, EGPRW and WONCA, the undergraduate departments played almost no role in any of them. Probably this reflected the need of those within universities to devote maximum effort to local pressures, but it also gave space to those outside the university system to pioneer different agendas. At the same time, individual academics and departments have contributed significantly to the development of general practice both as a clinical and as an academic discipline worldwide.

### General practice or public health?

The third tension has been that between the disciplines of general practice and public health. At one level, this has been an issue within universities. Although nearly all emerging departments of general practice required the patronage of departments of public health to grow, achieving independence from them thereafter was an inevitable evolutionary step. The tension between the emphasis of general practice on the needs of individual patients and that of public health on population medicine and the organisation of health services generally has been the public face of this dilemma, but the reluctance of departments of general practice to be seen merely as facilities for data collection for the epidemiological studies of others has been equally important. Now the emphasis is changing again, with universities wanting to merge small departments into larger ones, and the present risk is that this will result in general practice research moving more into disease-centred rather than patient-centred enquiry. This trend has already become evident in the 2008 RAE where the separate identity of general practice research has been greatly diminished by its re-positioning within other units of assessment in many universities, materially threatening the longer term future of general practice as an independent clinical discipline within medical schools.

Within the NHS, current initiatives to restructure general practice services reflect a shifting NHS emphasis towards public health agendas which may be quite different from the agendas of consulting patients.[8] In parallel, the increasingly frequent renaming of general practice as primary care warns of the possibility that general practice may in future not be a general practitioner led service.

## A second generation

Academic general practice looks very different in 2010 as compared to the 1970s. The renaming in 2000 of the discipline's scientific body from the AUDGP to the SAPC captured appropriately both the timing and the nature of what has almost amounted to a 'paradigm shift' in the discipline's profile. The discipline is now significantly more professional. Staff are much better trained in research methods, and the wide network of well briefed and supervised teaching general practices provides an enviable base for clinical teaching. The disciplinary spread is much wider than it was, although few of today's medical staff have had the depth of experience of full-time service practice that most of their predecessors had.

Academic general practice has had a challenging sixty-year lifespan. Its impact on the culture of medical schools has been visibly successful; its impact on the culture of service general practice has been harder to judge. In both spheres progress has been complicated (often unnecessarily) by issues of clinical and academic credibility, ownership of professional territory, and disciplinary identity. Many groups with differing agendas have been and still are competing for influence.

If academic general practice – whether by that name or as academic primary care (or even perhaps under some new name that better reflects other endangered elements of its original parent clinical discipline such as continuity and comprehensiveness of care) – is to continue to make a distinctive contribution in the future, it must be doubly sure of its contemporary identity and equally clear about its future aims.

*John Howie*

(This appendix is based on a presentation given at the sixtieth anniversary celebrations of the Edinburgh University Department of General Practice in Edinburgh during November 2008. The original version was published as Howie John G.R., 'Academic general practice – reflections on a 60-year journey', *Br J Gen Pract*, 60, 2010: 620–3. We gratefully acknowledge the editor's permission to reproduce it here.)

## Notes

1. Collings J.S., 'General practice in England today: a reconnaissance,' *Lancet*, i, 1950: 55–85.
2. Horder J.P., 'Developments in other countries', in *General Practice under the National Health Service, 1948–1997*, Clarendon Press, London, 1998, p. 256.

3. McWhinney I.R., 'General practice as an academic discipline', *Lancet*, i, 1966: 419–23.
4. Richardson I.M., 'The value of a university department of general practice', *BMJ*, iv, 1975: 740–2.
5. Pereira Gray D.J. (ed.), *Forty Years On: The Story of the First Forty Years of the Royal College of General Practitioners*, London: RCGP, 1992.
6. Howie J.G.R., Hannay D.R. and Stevenson J.S.K., *The Mackenzie Report: General Practice in the Medical Schools of the United Kingdom – 1986*, Edinburgh, University of Edinburgh, 1986.
7. Royal College of General Practitioners, *The Future General Practitioner: Learning and Teaching*, London, RCGP, 1972.
8. Howie J.G.R., Metcalfe D.H.H. and Walker J.H., 'The state of general practice – not all for the better', *BMJ*, 336, 2008: 1310.

## Further reading

Loudon I., Horder J. and Webster C., *General Practice Under the National Health Service 1948–1997*, Clarendon Press, London, 1998.

## Appendix 4  And Finally . . .

The last decade has been a time of considerable change for academic primary care. At the turn of the millennium, where the main departmental stories end, there was a record number of stand-alone departments of primary care/general practice across the UK and a recently reinvigorated workforce thanks to pump priming monies from the 1997 Primary Care Research and Development Review. There was also a palpable step change in the depth, quality and international standing of British primary care research, reflected in the results of the 2008 RAE.[1] Indeed a recent benchmarking exercise comparing the volume and quality of original primary care research published by six countries with well-established academic primary care found that UK primary care researchers ranked first or second in every citation metric examined. The establishment of the NIHR school for primary care research in England in 2006 also reflected both the priority given to and the excellence of academic primary care research. The school comprises the eight leading academic centres for primary care research in England and has access to £4 million each year to fund cutting-edge collaborative research. There are similar though less-funded schools in Scotland and Wales. Primary care academics have also been instrumental in continuing to develop and deliver community-based undergraduate medical education, which now makes up a large part of every medical school's curriculum.

However, we are now entering more uncertain times. The 'credit crunch' felt in every home in the land has also affected the academic community and in future it is likely we will be asked to do more with less. Whilst some academics may be sheltered somewhat by their position within national schools, all will have to work harder to maintain their productivity and excellence. Academic primary care also faces challenges in terms of its workforce. Only one in 225 general practitioners in the UK are clinical academics compared to approximately one in sixteen consultants in all hospital specialities, and the current number of academic general practice training posts is insufficient to sustain existing capacity.[2] Indeed the membership of SAPC is 'top heavy', an inverted pyramid, with far fewer lecturers and fellows than senior posts. A less obvious cause for concern is the emerging emphasis on primary care trials as the dominant methodology. Indeed the PCRN achieves around 30 per cent of all accruals across the NIHR Clinical Research Network. However an unintended consequence of positioning clinical trials as the most natural infrastructure for research within a primary care population laboratory is the devaluing of multi-method research in or by primary care.[3] Preparation for the Research Excellence Framework is also having an impact on primary care research. Many UK medical schools are being restructured into larger mainly bench to bedside disease-focused research groupings. Stand-alone departments of primary care are slowly disappearing, subsumed strategically into larger departmental groupings. Whilst it could be argued that a disease- rather than a context-specific focus for research is a sign of disciplinary maturity, my personal worry is that the unique generalist nature of primary care activity and service delivery will be lost.

Of course times of great change offer opportunities. The recent White Paper[4] has catapulted primary care onto the centre of the NHS stage. A high quality mixed-method patient-centred context-specific primary care evidence base is needed to underpin commissioning decisions. Multidisciplinary departments of primary care understand how to provide this and evaluate the consequences of changes to service delivery. The need to focus on this 'second translational gap' (between research and health care delivery) was of course highlighted as a key part of the future research agenda for primary care long before the White Paper was published.[5]

But practical strategies are required as well as heartfelt rhetoric. Academic primary care can only continue to 'punch above its weight' if the brightest and best are recruited. This means a concerted and continued effort to ensure the value of evidence-based medicine and its teaching as part of the undergraduate and postgraduate curriculum, and ensuring that primary care personnel continue to be co-producers of that evidence. Five-year training for general practitioners that includes a research component would also help. We need to work with the NIHR, with deaneries, the RCGP and perhaps pharmaceutical companies to create new posts that attract and develop new researchers and teachers rather than simply recycling current talent! If more practices were involved in research, perhaps through Research Ready (the RCGP online research accreditation scheme), research-active general practitioners could more readily act as mentors for registrars, normalising the notion of scholarship in everyday clinical practice. Non-medical primary care researchers also need to feel that academic departments of primary care are their natural home. This can only happen if career pathways are clear, fair, flexible and above all equitable with medical colleagues.

This book has clearly demonstrated the battles our forefathers fought and won to establish academic primary care as a substantive and valid academic discipline. A new generation of multidisciplinary primary care academics now need to rise to the challenges described and ensure that the UK continues to be the international trailblazer.

*Helen Lester (Chair SAPC)*

## Notes

1. Howe A., 'UK general practice is the best in the world', *RCGP News*, March 2009.
2. Medical Schools Council, *Staffing Levels of Medical Clinical Academics in UK Medical Schools at 31 July 2008*, Medical Schools Council, London, 2008.
3. Shaw S. and Greenhalgh T., 'Best research – for what? Best health – for whom? A critical exploration of primary care research using discourse analysis', *Soc Sci Med*, 66, 2008: 2506–19.
4. Department of Health, *Equity and Excellence: Liberating the NHS*, London, 2010.
5. The Academy for Medical Sciences, *Research in General Practice: Bringing Innovation into Patient Care*, Workshop Report, 2009.

# Index